CW00495096

DISCLAIMER

This text is primarily aimed at **UK Activity Coordinators.**

The publisher and author provide this book and its contents on an 'as is' basis and make no representation or warranties of any kind with respect to this book or its contents. The publisher and author disclaim all such representations and warranties and assume no responsibility for errors, inaccuracies, omissions, or any inconsistencies herein. You understand this book is not intended as a substitute for your own Company's Codes of Practice and Policies and Procedures. The use of this book implies your acceptance of this disclaimer. The publisher and author make no guarantees concerning the level of success you may experience by following the advice and strategies contained in this book, and you accept that results may differ for each individual.

The publisher and author have made every effort to ensure the information in this book was correct at the time of going to press and do not assume and hereby disclaim any liability to any party for loss, damage or disruption caused by errors or omissions. Any advice or recommendations are made without guarantee on the part of the author or publisher. The author and publisher disclaim any liability in connection with the use of this information. The information in this book is provided for general informational and educational purposes only. The author makes no representations or warranties, express or implied, about the completeness, accuracy, reliability, suitability, or availability with respect to the information, products, services, or related graphics contained in this book for any purposes. Any use of the information contained in this book is at your own risk. The author of this book disclaims liability for any loss or damage suffered by any person as a result of the information or content in this book.

Published by

Blue Giraffe Publishing

*"May all your headaches be solved with creativity and a little
sparkle"*

Activity Handbook

All you want to know but were afraid to ask

CREATED BY

ALISON MOORE

COVER DESIGN & ILLUSTRATIONS BY

CHARLOTTE MOORE

Dementia Person-centred Activity Specialist

Award Winner

CQC "Outstanding"

CONTENTS

Chapter 1   Introduction

Meaningful person-centred activities in a care home setting are an integral part of the overall care package. Creating activities for your residents is only just a part of your role, making them person-centred to each resident can be challenging but rewarding.

- But how do we achieve a person-centred approach rather than just organise activities that we think residents will like?
- Once organised, how do we deliver them in such a way that they are meaningful to every person in our care?
- A large part of our job is recording responses, likes, dislikes as well as personality traits in line with company policies and procedures: how do we find time to fit it all in?

This book is a guide to helping you build the foundations for a smoother working life and covering the groundwork in a time-effective manner, with the bonus your files are in place when the inspectors arrive.

This book is aimed at both experienced practitioners wishing to introduce procedures that comply with today's protocol, and those new to the profession.

Always remember;

> *'If it's not written down, it didn't happen!'*

But who am I to be writing this?

Having dived in at the deep end in a Dementia and ABI nursing home that specialised in mid to late-stage dementia and was the preferred provider in the locality for those with challenging behaviour, I rapidly learnt about person-centred care and activities, along with anti-psychotics and challenging behaviour: it was an eye-opener.

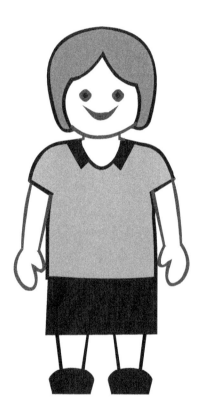

My CPD[continuing professional development] includes a QCF in Activities: not just for dementia residents but covering mental health and general care home activities. As well as writing a training manual for staff involvement and a workbook for work placement students, I also have qualifications in Business Start-Up and Management as well as being a Customer Care Assessor. I took to the job like the proverbial duck to water and was proud to be an important part of the team who attained 4/5 outstanding from the CQC. That's in the top 3% of the UK: something I will always be proud of.

Whilst gaining experience on the job I felt the staff needed a reference point for enhancing the life enrichment of the residents as they were, in part responsible for facilitating the enrichment activities I devised. I wrote a short manual that I then used as a basis of enrichment for the section they worked in. This encouraged the staff to share the workload fairly and also to realise that they were already doing meaningful activities without realising it.

 We also accommodated students on work experience from the local college who came with no criteria on how they were to widen their scope whilst they were present. I wrote a work experience handbook that they kept on completion and would help form part of their course work.

So why write this book?

What did surprise me once I started the role was the lack of information that was written down about how to manage the role effectively and to document it in the correct way for the authorities to monitor what we were doing: the CQC [Care Quality Commission].

I scoured the internet for advice and books that I could gain information from and found there was very little.

The majority of publications concentrate on activities, mostly activities for the cognitive and able. As our home is mostly mid to late-stage dementia, these activity books, although good, were not suitable for our residents. None of them prepares you for the mountain of evidence that is required, and how you can make it easier for yourself for when the inspectors call!

After not only surviving the CQC visit but impressing them with the structure we have in place, I wanted to share how to document and organise life so that you are not run ragged and end up doing work at home. That is just a no-no.

This won't be a rule book, but more to get your creative juices flowing differently so that you can use my experience and ideas to improve your work flow.

Where do we begin?

The world of activities is evolving into a much more prominent and important role within a care home setting. In fact, it is coming to be the lynch-pin of a home for many reasons; whether the residents are cognitive and able-bodied or have severe dementia, so we must endeavour to get it right. The governing bodies of countries all over the world now look far more closely at what we create than they ever have before. The creation of suitable activities for our residents not only allows them to lead enriched lives but also can reduce aggressive episodes and reduce the need for anti-psychotic drugs. As for the staff; it makes their job a lot easier too.

 The Activity Staff roles are now being treated as more important than ever and respect is growing for the valuable work we do: so, let's get it right!

But is the word 'activities' the right word for our job role? In this day and age, I think not. We do not just provide things for people to do such as bingo and colouring, our role is much more complex. We are there to get to know residents and to provide life enrichment for them 'individually' which is a much harder and in-depth task. We try to enrich the lives of our residents with things that mean something to them personally and that will stimulate their abilities. With our help, residents live a fuller and more settled life and if we get it right, the support workers have fewer negative behaviours to deal with too.

When we get it right, the ripples go through the whole home enhancing everyone's day. But we have to sow the first seeds for a great home to grow.

The journey is as important as the destination

Chapter 2   **Being Person-centred**

What is being person-centred and how do we practice it?

It surprises me that all over the world there are still care facilities that do things that are task-orientated, especially when it comes to activity planning. Thankfully, most companies who provide care home activities have a changed attitude to their daily care of residents. Activities for those residents is now seen as a key part of their day in the home.

Insisting person-centred care is delivered throughout a home can be met with confusion. Staff either don't want to change from what they already do, or are already person-centred and didn't realise it.

The fear of change in any profession is ever-present so can we describe the difference easily?

Let's look at these two scenarios.

Situation 1:

Lizzie is 84 years old and has been living in a Dementia Care Home for 3 years. The staff get her up at 7.30 am every day even though she is sleepy and she lashes out during personal care. She is given cereals for breakfast and if she doesn't eat it by 8.15 am it is taken away.

Lizzie spends the morning hungry all bar a cup of coffee and a biscuit at 11 am. The coffee goes cold as she prefers tea. Staff scold her as they replace it with juice. She doesn't like juice either.

At lunchtime, Lizzie is taken to an unlaid kitchen table to eat and a plate, piled high with food, is placed in front of her and the staff move on to dish up for the next person. Lizzie slowly works her way around the plate but 30 minutes later it is removed and dessert put in front of her. Somewhat confused, Lizzie tries the pudding but finds it hard to break the pastry crust of the apple pie with her spoon; she just doesn't have the strength any more.

The staff assume she is not hungry and remove the dish before escorting her to the lounge where she is sat in front of a loud TV for the afternoon. Teatime is a repeat scenario of lunch before Lizzie is whisked off to bed before the night staff arrive on shift at 8 pm. Lizzie once more lashes out at staff as she doesn't want to go to bed. Drugs are administered to calm her down and her bedroom door shut as staff leave, and she is still hungry.

Situation 2:

Betty is 79 and enjoys a lie in. The staff keep their eye on her until she is awake. They then put her favourite music on and chat with her about how beautiful the morning is and serve her favourite breakfast of fresh fruit and yoghurt as she sits up in bed. They take time to sit and chat with Betty as she eats her breakfast and, when she is ready, the staff explain the personal care they are about to do. They ask Betty what she would like to wear today, holding outfits in front of her so that she can choose.

Once Betty is dressed, she is given the choice of where she would like to sit today. Betty chooses to go by the window so that she can watch people walking by. Betty enjoys waving to the school children as they walk past and staff sit with her whilst filling in their paperwork, sometimes chatting over a cup of tea.
Betty is asked where she would like to sit to eat her lunch. She chooses to sit at the dining table which looks very pretty with a tablecloth, napkins and cutlery that had been laid by another resident.

Betty is given a choice of what to eat and chooses sausages and mashed potatoes. Knowing Betty struggles to cut meat, the staff asks her if she would like to have her sausages cut into pieces. Betty smiles warmly and nods her head. Betty is a slow eater and likes to chat with Edith over lunch, they have formed a great friendship.

When Betty indicates she has finished eating she asks to go to the lounge window again and Edith sits with her so they can chat and watch the world go by. Over tea and biscuits in the afternoon a member of staff asks which book they would like to have read aloud.

After teatime whilst the staff are helping other residents to bed, Betty and Edith enjoy watching their favourite game show and then the news. Betty enjoys knowing what is going on in the world and will chat about it to staff. When Betty is ready for bed the staff take her to her room where she watches her favourite soap whilst having a cup of hot chocolate. A staff member joins her with her cup of tea. Betty is happy and relaxed.

Which of these two ladies do you connect with most? Ideally Betty; who is receiving person-centred care which allows Betty to decide what she wants and when she wants it. The attention to Betty's needs ensures that she continues to make as many choices as she can in her life.

By having control over her day, Betty is a more relaxed and happier person. The staff being person-centred as part of their daily routine helps everyone have a better day.

As for Lizzie's day: well, it stands a good chance that she is not happy at all and instead of her medication being decreased, the staff will increase it to cope with her 'behaviours'. In Lizzie's home the staff are going through their daily routine without person-centred thought for the residents. What effect does this type of attitude have? Would the residents be happy and cared for? Do you think they would be active when they can be or would they become morose being stuck in front of the TV every day? What mood would they be in as no one is taking the time to talk to them?

Most residents wouldprobably feel agitated and upset that they are neglected and misunderstood. This could have the knock-on effect of the residents going off-baseline and then give staff added issues in settling them down again.

Always remember that when someone goes off baseline it can take hours before they are back in their happy place. Of course, some homes would administer drugs to keep residents calm, but the majority of residents receiving person-centred care will be on reduced antipsychotic drugs. Those labelled as violent often settle well into a person-centred community with rarely any further signs of violence.

What is important is to ensure that everything you devise and put in place is person-centred. So, what is the difference between being person-centred and being task orientated? I see so many people having a daily calendar that is rammed from 9 am to 7 pm with activities every 30 minutes that I have visions of crashing walking frames with residents piled in a heap! Thinking about these busy and active days I do wonder how person-centred the activities are and how you manage to get all these things jammed in. I know that in some of the USA residential homes, there are specifics that require these full-day calendars, but is it beneficial to residents?

A task-driven calendar only works on paper: tick box exercises so to speak. It has little benefit for the majority of the residents and will only work to a large extent in homes that are for the elderly who are fit and able.

This kind of calendar fails to produce the right results for residents in homes where illnesses are the prime reason for them being there. Their lack of ability to complete the tasks and the packed schedule sets residents up to fail. This can lead to poor mental and physical health and an increase in adverse behaviours: not something we want to encourage. Whereas a tailored, carefully planned person-centred calendar has much more scope for residents to be empowered during activities. But if you are new to the role, how will you know what is what?

Task Orientated

- Your calendar is jam-packed with activities at allotted times.
- Each activity starts and finishes on time

- Activities are random and things we **think** people want to do
- Activities are repetitive

What would a typical task-driven day look like?

6.30-9 am	Residents up and given breakfast in the dining room
9-10 am	First activity, card making
10-11 am	Singing
11-12 noon	Bingo
12-1 pm	Lunch from the menu in the dining room
1-2 pm	Art therapy
2-3 pm	Gardening
3-4 pm	Bible Study
4-5 pm	Afternoon tea from the menu in the dining room
5-6 pm	Chair Yoga
6-7 pm	Flower arranging
7 onwards	TV time and Bedtime

What would a typical *person-centred* day look like?

- The calendar is selective and flexible
- Activities have meaning and are not expected to have a full attendance
- Start and finish times are for the most part open-ended
- Fewer planned activities
- Random on the spot activities

AM	Residents rise and are asked what they would like to wear, where they would like to have breakfast and where they would like to eat it
AM	Staff spend time with residents chatting, giving hand massages or utilising the Activity Box [see further in the book] which has various items inside like playing cards, dominoes, books, CD's, pens and paper
Lunchtime	Residents are offered a choice of food and asked where they would like to eat it.
PM	Organised activity that will have been carefully thought out with the residents' choices in mind
PM	Afternoon snacks and drinks, mocktails [non-alcoholic cocktails] and fruit tasting
PM	Music and interaction with sing-a-long, dancing
PM	Teatime. Residents choice of food from the menu
PM	Relax with staff chatting, watching residents' choices of TV programmes. Preparing people for bed at a time of their choosing.

How do these compare with what you are doing?

Yes, certain tasks have to be completed at certain times such as meal times.

But to be person-centred there has to be flexibility to the day. Think about how you like to live your own life especially when you are not at work. A lie in of a Sunday morning, choosing what and where to have breakfast: going out even for brunch and bypassing breakfast.

In our daily lives, **WE** choose what **WE** want to do and when we want to do it.

Imagine if you were told day in day out what you were eating. You were woken and dressed at 7 am every day with no choice to have that lovely lie in. This lack of choice can lead to a person being institutionalised and to make matters worse, they can become unresponsive, aggressive and bored, leading to possible illness, negative behaviours and potentially an increase in medication to calm them down.

Living a person-centred lifestyle stimulates residents, they stay awake longer as they are less likely to be bored, and the need for anti-psychotic drugs can often be reduced with a Doctor's consultation.

The other massive bonus to running activities in a person-centred way is that with residents happy, there are fewer incidents to report and staff have a happier time at work. The whole atmosphere of the home improves because residents are happier.

With the right outlook, days are easier for staff too. Happy residents make for happy staff and less paperwork. This has a ripple effect throughout the home and when families visit, it passes through to them too. It's a win-win situation.

To create a programme of activities we have to know our residents. You will have comprehensive care plans that will give you a balanced idea of the resident as well as spending time with them.

I will cover care plans in more depth, later on. Currently, I'm expecting you to have good ones so you can work from them and start to get yourself organised.

- Medical Pages
  Find a suitable time to sit with nursing staff so that you can understand what the drugs the resident is taking does for them, whether they can have behavioural side effects, any underlying conditions

- Lifestyle Pages
  One-page profiles, lifestyle pages and 'This is Me' [see template]

- Dietary
  Important to find out about allergies and intolerances, likes and dislikes

- Activities
  Documentation from the previous coordinator about what works and what doesn't. If it didn't work for them, always try it again.

- The resident
  The most important part is to build up your own picture of each resident. This will take time and chatting with staff is another important tool for creating that overall picture as well as chatting to the resident.

Talking with the resident's family and getting to know them is important. Often, they are our only way of getting to know our new resident. It is also important for families to see that we are interested in and doing the best for the resident.

Families are becoming more knowledgeable about the operation of care homes so engaging with them is valuable for them and us. You will get some that think that their family member deserves the utmost priority, so you have to be kind but firm in your response.

It's like starting with blank pieces of a jigsaw puzzle that start to become colourful the more you engage with the residents. It takes time to gather a lot of information on each resident so add elements as and when you find out information; even the smallest detail.

Always remember that we need to live in their world and treat them with dignity and respect.

Care plans become your best friends once you get your head around them, providing they have been completed in line with Policies and Procedures set down by the company you work for.

There's a lot of medical information that you can leave until later but it's always worth getting a nurse to explain what effect drugs can have on people. To begin with, this section of care plans can muddy the waters of what you want to achieve. Don't try to read too many in one go as you'll get muddled. The technique that worked for me was to sit with a resident whilst reading their care plan or have a chat with them before or after reading it.

ALWAYS ask families and residents if they can complete a 'This is Me' booklet [see Templates]: the more information you get the easier planning activities for them will be. Especially include the little quirks they have, why they say certain names, refer to certain things, what they love or hate and what foods they prefer and how they like them prepared. In an ideal world, the booklet will be full of detail and hopefully useful photographs once completed as these can be used in memory chats.

If you are really lucky, the previous AC or care staff will have written an enrichment plan based on this document. This should focus on all areas of enrichment tailored to the specific resident. This is not something that can be created overnight and you will need the assistance of care staff to help build up the detail and the specific activities to enrich the resident's life.

You can plan general activities from the start and then tailor them more over time. Some activities might not work but don't give up on them if you think they are a good idea. Park it for a while then try it again. You never know what reaction you might get.

One other thing to remember is to document your activity interaction with each resident. If you haven't already got a company plan for this then there is one in the template section you can use and adapt.

You need to record WHEN something was offered to the resident, WHAT they did and the OUTCOME. You may find that some residents will always refuse to do any form of arranged activity. Instead of ignoring this, it is important to document that it has been refused.

Here's a sample of filling in a sheet:

INTERACTION RECORD SHEET

NAME..... Peter Smith .... ROOM No;...7c....

ACTIVITY UNDERTAKEN/~~DECLINED~~ 1:1.×. GROUP.... DATE.2/10/2020

> Balloon Tennis

OUTCOME

> Peter was not wanting to join in a group session so we took some balloons to his room for him to interact on a 1:1 basis. He soon asked for the blue balloon and was passing it too and fro. Peter was smiling and laughing.

LED BY....Sue.F...

ACTIVITY UNDERTAKEN/~~DECLINED~~ 1:1.... GROUP. × DATE.5/10/2020

> Baking Cup Cakes

OUTCOME

> Peter enjoyed cooking at home when his wife Janice was alive so he was eager to help in mixing and putting into the cupcake cases. He also enjoyed sharing them with other residents after their evening meal. He said that Janice would be proud as he licked cake mix off his fingers.

LED BY....Sue F..

Why do Person-Centred activities work?

As you can see from the previous examples, we are much more aware that the quality of life residents in care have is important. Residents can lead a rich and fulfilling life rather than being bored and sat in front of a TV all day.

By taking the time to get to know the residents we enrich their lives by creating activities that suit their needs. It's difficult to start fresh doing the research but it is so rewarding to see the pleasure that your activities can bring.

As an example, I discovered that by reading the Care Plans, a large sector of our residents went to church all their lives. I contacted the local diocese and arranged for a vicar to come in and deliver a service. I was incredibly nervous and wondered how many of the 56 residents would turn up especially as about 85% would need wheelchair assistance. I was aghast when the staff brought 95% of residents to the service and about 25% of those had their partners with them too.

We spilt out of our room and into the reception. The joy it brought to everyone was something really special. It then became a regular occurrence with staff only too happy to assist as they took a lot from it too. That happy feeling lasted longer than the hour for those residents. It had a positive effect on them for the next day or longer. This led to a more receptive and alert resident.

If this can happen with one person-centred activity imagine what it's like when your whole activity calendar is person-centred.

Something that can be forgotten about is how you talk with the residents. I've heard people talk to them like they were in nursery school or hardly talk to them at all.

Residents must be spoken to respectfully. Put yourself in their shoes: you are living in a place called home that isn't what you think of as home. You are away from family, you have people doing personal care that you find invades your privacy but you are unable to do it yourself and the staff talk to you in an unfitting way because you are unable to express yourself in the way you used to. How would that make you feel?

- Don't patronise, don't assume and don't treat people like babies. Call people by their name, show them respect and explain what is happening at all times even if you've said it 100 times before. Do it with a smile and a thought for what they are experiencing.
- Be patient and wait for answers.
- Look at your body language to see how it reflects on the residents and what they pick up on.
- Be aware of those with sensory impairments. If Doris is deaf and choses not to wear a hearing aid because the noise from others distorts the sound, position yourself so that she can lip read. If Joe has sight impairment ensure he sits next to you so that you can guide things into his hands and you can explain what you are doing. He can feel the pot of soil and run it through his fingers and smell it. If George has arthritis in his fingers, help him to hold a smaller, more suitable pot or plant in a mug that he can grab the handle of.

- Don't ever set anyone up to fail. Don't set goals that residents will be unable to reach. Try to keep the activity and length of the session open-ended and if someone wants to leave before the others, that's fine. They will have done all they wanted to do and maybe just want to go watch their favourite TV programme. It's OK so don't see it as a failure on your part or theirs.

- Don't take over! Just because Rose is being slower to do the activity than the rest of the group, resist the temptation to bring her up to speed. Let Rose enjoy doing what she is doing in her way. Again, encourage her in what she is doing and help if required but don't rush. Always remember it's Rose who this activity is for not you.

- Being person-centred involves a lot of change in our behaviours too. It can take time to fully develop this and we are not perfect. You will find that over time this meaningful way of being will flip into your personal life and you will be more understanding of people in general. It's a good thing all around.

Communication

Talking with residents may not be the only way for you to communicate. You may need to use sight language, whiteboards or a set of pictorial cards to make sure you are understood and that they can express to you their needs and mood.

Getting to know which resident need to lip read or who need extra time to process something you have said to them is paramount and should be documented in their care plan. Keep any questions simple and to the point using only two options at a time and keep at eye level but don't overcrowd them. Have open body language and be aware of theirs.

Language barriers can crop up if a resident is of foreign descent or has reverted to speaking their mother tongue if they have dementia. Use cards in both languages for them to read or learn a little of their language. Never ignore someone because you don't feel comfortable communicating, try and you will succeed.

Chapter 3   How creative do we have to be?

All of us have a difficult job to do whichever sector of the care home business we work in. Yes, those with cognitive ability and physical ability are easier to engage in a wider range of activities but that in itself involves you stretching your mind in being creative.

Bingo is an activity that crops up regularly, but sadly I hear more negatives than positives. Issues with the caller being too slow or too quick, people hogging the best prizes, no funds to buy prizes, people wanting better prizes, arguing amongst residents, the list is endless. A word of advice; add bingo at your peril and have a clear plan beforehand on how you will run it and distribute prizes if you give prizes at all.

It's the taking part that's important to make it a fun experience. Change numbers to animals, cartoon characters or shapes, make it a social gathering with tea and cakes. Change it up to keep it fresh.

Once you have studied your residents you begin to mentally put them into groups for shared interests. It's a good idea when studying care plans to start lists of group activities and which people like them. This simple table below helps to clearly show groups for activities that you can utilise over other topics too.

GARDENING	MUSIC	ARTS & CRAFTS
Bert	Bert	Susan
Nancy	Phyllis	Nancy
Joe	Susan	Pat
Roger	Michael	Janice
	Steve	Cath
	Clive	Roger
	June	
	David	

By keeping lists, you can create activities to suit small or large groups and be mindful of where you locate the activity and how many staff you will need to assist with it.

Music is loved by the majority so you can have listening sessions to their choice of music or watching videos, live entertainment, karaoke or sing-a-long.

Gardening can be done indoors and out. Planting seeds, weeding, a walk enjoying and discussing the grounds.

Arts and Crafts are endless from making cards to Christmas trimmings. Although if you use glitter you will be finding it in your hair for weeks!

All of the group activities can be a good social interaction for residents to meet people they don't normally see. Adding in tea and cakes is a good ice breaker.

With any activity always remember it's the taking part that counts not the completion of the project or doing it 'right'.

You may have residents with different abilities, so you can split the activity into sections so that Bert sorts and opens the seed packets, Nancy adds compost to pots so Bert can pop the seeds in and Joe fetches the watering can, fills with water and waters the pots. Each has fulfilled a part of a whole without pressure on them to do things they can no longer do.

Some will instinctively know what to do and some will be hesitant. You may well need to sit people in such a way that you can work more closely with one or two people while you keep an eye on the group. It is important not to segregate anyone whilst doing this as they may feel isolated. You may also find that you have a resident who is happy to assist someone less able. If you are working alone with a group you do need to have eyes in the back of your head to see what everyone is doing but if you can ask a member of staff to assist for even 15 minutes it's a big help. Some homes have dedicated 1:1 allocation so if you can include that resident and carer in a group it gives you extra support.

Have a couple of extra little tasks to one side so that if you are still working with one or two residents you can add something onto the table for others to do, such as tearing up bits of newspaper to go into the compost, counting the pots that have been planted or writing labels for them. Anything that you think will suit their ability whilst you are busy with the others in the group.

If the seeds get mixed up, does it matter?

If the soil goes on the floor, does it matter?

All that matters is that residents have enjoyed themselves doing something they enjoy. It's very hard not to focus on the completed project. It's also hard not to rush people along because it's time for lunch or your break. Explain to them that it is time for their lunch if they'd like it and that they can return later if they wish.

You will always have people who do not want to engage with groups but they may be happy to sit on the side-lines listening to the chatter or watching what is going on. Allow them their space but ensure you engage with them throughout the activity. They may at some point decide to join in or they may just doze off to sleep. It's their choice but what they are doing is making that choice for themselves so you do need to document what you offered and how they did or didn't engage.

Your creativity will increase as you become more confident in the role, it takes time to settle in and develop your calendar of events. If things are popular, repeat them every few weeks or once a month. If something doesn't go down well, have a look at the structure, see if it can be improved and then try again. If it doesn't work it doesn't matter. Move onto the next activity.

It's always handy to keep a file of activities for reference with notes of what worked and what didn't. It's especially handy if you are off work and staff can dip in to add something to the day. Activities are always evolving as residents come and go and their abilities change, so you need to keep yourself aware of that.

With a 1:1 activity, you can usually adapt a group activity to a 1:1 or 1:2 setting. You can take planting seeds to someone who is room bound and conduct the activity there. The resident may do as much or as little as they like or just be happy watching you plant a seed for them. Encourage them to be involved in the watering and ask staff to ensure they show the resident the pot daily to see it start to grow and watch its progress.

NOTES

I spent the first 3 months getting to know the residents and staff and creating first weekly activities then moved onto monthly. I was constantly chasing my tail with weekly calendars so I took the leap to monthly and found life was much easier.

Chapter 4   **Care Planning**

'If it's not written down, it didn't happen'

Although the Activity Coordinator isn't responsible for the medical sections of the care plan, it is expected that you will be responsible for the enrichment/activity/lifestyle section. Again, you may be lucky enough to step into the shoes of someone thorough and organised but this can be rare.

We all think differently so 'organised' to one person is far from it to others! It's also not a bad idea to start with a clean slate so that you can put your stamp on things and you are also looking at residents with fresh eyes.

What if you are new to the role and haven't a clue what to do? You may have been told about the aforementioned paperwork as well as creating and delivering activities to residents, but how? I would suggest in the beginning you need to be on good terms with all staff and residents. Listen to them all, you'll hear a lot of stories about past activity coordinators as well as getting nuggets of great information about residents and fellow staff.

If you are lucky enough to have assistants, arrange regular meetings with them so that they can pass on their knowledge to you. This will not only be valuable to you but also ensures that they feel part of the team.

At this point, it is very important to listen and take notes. Go everywhere with a notebook, I can't stress how important this is. I'd also suggest that you spend the last 15-30 minutes of your day jotting down things you have learnt and ideas you have had plus any questions that crop up both for you and staff. For at least the first few weeks your head will be full of so much stuff that unless you write it down you won't sleep. I mean that positively as you will be buzzing! This new habit will allow you to relax when you leave work and also prepares you for the next day.

Other things to write down are the things that made you smile during the day and the things you think you can improve on. Also be self-aware: document things that make you feel uncomfortable and that you need to improve on to make yourself better at your job. [Personal Reflections Template.] Working in care in any capacity is a continuous self-learning process and you will become aware of things about yourself that you never knew.

In general, your role will involve you organising activities within the home and outside. If you are fortunate enough to have a minibus you may be required to be the driver for this too. Try to ensure this task is shared with others so that you don't become a general dogsbody going to collect anything and everything. It can be far too easy to get sucked into another role when your role alone is demanding enough!

Always ensure you follow your company's policy on how many staff should be on the minibus per resident. Being alone is a definite no-no, you never know what could happen whilst you are trying to concentrate on the road ahead.

Another role not to get sucked into is assisting with personal care. Unless it's in your contract, avoid it. If you are doing it right, you will not have time to do a second job as well as your own. Plus, once you have done it once, you will be called upon time after time to step in for absent staff and then that's your whole shift swallowed up!

Set your boundaries and stick to your job description. Be polite and firm from the start but do it nicely so no one gets offended. OK, we all help each other out as that's being part of a team but you really can help out too much: I can't emphasise that enough. Otherwise, you will soon become exhausted and not have enough time to commit to your role, standards will slip and it will be hard to claw yourself back to where you were.

The care plan for a resident as we know is a living document, so it needs to be well written with as much detail as possible. Try not to get distracted by the nursing aspect of a care plan other than to utilise the relevant elements that will give the bigger picture of the resident. As I said previously, it is important to understand the effects that certain drugs have on the resident, whether they will be drowsy and how long after taking them etc.

It depends on how your company records data and to the regulations in your country as to how complete they are. If you are fortunate enough to be stepping into the shoes of someone competent in their role, then it will be easy to follow suit and just update plans accordingly. But what I hear from many newcomers to the role is that there is no evidence of activity records and they do not know where to start.

What did the family provide you when their resident came to stay?

Photographs   With any photographs it's helpful if you can get the family to write down who is in the pictures. Photocopy them and add the names. These can then take the form of a reminiscence book that can be used for conversation. Some can be put on the wall of the resident's room so that they have familiar faces and places around them.

This is Me   A very important element to creating the whole picture of the resident. *[Template Section]*.

It's worth building up a good relationship with the family members. Often there are things that they won't remember to put down in 'This is Me' but they will recall when relaxed and having a chat with you. It's important that they feel comfortable to be in your company and build up trust in the activities you are devising for their loved ones. They will often come up with some good ideas and/or bring things in that can be used within the home.

Having a good relationship with families means a lot for them too. You become their point of contact as the 'middleman' between their loved one and the management. They will often talk to you and are generally happy to work with you on any fundraising or home projects. Their lives are difficult too, and they are also part of the home and the care we deliver to their loved ones. It makes them feel good to participate in things at the home and assist or join in external activities.

Once you have gathered this information how do you put it together in a meaningful document? You need to create a 'Meaningful Living Plan' *[templates]* for the resident. I know you will probably groan that I'm adding in more paperwork but this can prove very effective when new staff come or an agency worker. It is a quick read for them to get to know the residents they are caring for.

At the top of the document should be the person's details, name, date of birth and a brief description of what the document is about.

For example, *'Helping John Smith to lead a fulfilling life'*. Also, include here details of the name the resident prefers to be called. It's quite common for someone to be referred to by another name entirely or have a preference for being called by an abbreviated version. There's nothing more annoying to family than someone who is used to being called Michael being referred to as Mike, Mick or Micky. Some can prefer to be called Mr Smith especially as staff are much younger than them and it shows respect for your elders.

Add the main details that say who John is: -

Family   John is married to Janet and they have three children Denise, Beth and George

                Denise is married to Philip and they have two children Stephen and Sophie

                Beth is single as is George

                John and Janet married in 1968

                John has two brothers William and Peter and a sister Susan who died in 1998

Homelife   John loved his garden and had a greenhouse where he liked to grow tomatoes and herbs which Janet would use for cooking

                John loved having pets, dogs were his favourite but he and Janet recently adopted two stray kittens

John had his favourite armchair by the window where he would read. John's family are bringing his chair in for him

John enjoyed driving and when the children were small, they would tour various parts of the country towing their caravan. In their later years, John and Janet bought a static caravan by the sea in Tenby

Hobbies	John loved reading books by Lee Child and John le Carré
	John also had a passion for motorbikes and enjoyed watching the moto GP on TV. He didn't like football but would happily watch motorsports
	John liked to read the newspaper before having his evening meal
Career	John was in the RAF for 12 years as an engineer
	After the RAF, John went on to start his own engineering company 'Smith & Son' which his son George now runs
Food	John enjoys a variety of food including Italian and Indian but not too hot. He is not a lover of plain food
	John dislikes cabbage and spinach
	John loves desserts especially anything with thick custard
Allergies	John is allergic to strawberries

Medical   John suffers from arthritis in his hands and is type 2
                 diabetic

Then move on to incorporating the eight dimensions of wellness: -
physical, mental, emotional, occupational, social, intellectual,
environmental, sensory and spiritual.

Physical   John can walk unaided for short distances but may
                 need a wheelchair for longer trips. Please check his
                 care plan before going on an outing

                 John enjoys going for rides in the country and out for
                 a cup of tea and a cake

Environmental

                 John likes his living space to be cosy with side lamps
                 rather than overhead lighting. John likes to have a
                 choice of books to read and music to listen to rather
                 than TV during the day. He likes to have plants on the
                 windowsill that he can tend

Emotional   John enjoys family visits especially when the family
                 look at photographs together

                 John can be tactile when he chooses and enjoys a hug
                 from people he knows

                 John responds well to happy, smiling faces

Occupational   John likes to be helpful. He used to keep the accounts
                 for the company so will like to do things where he
                 can organise paperwork

	John enjoyed gardening so may like to help in planting seeds or plants
Social	John likes to be in the company of those he knows but doesn't like large groups as they can be noisy
	John does enjoy going out for walks and to go for meals
	John prefers to see what is going on before joining in
Intellectual	John is an intelligent man who enjoys stimulating conversation
	John likes to read the newspaper, preferably The Telegraph
Spiritual	John was brought up Christian and he and his wife Janet often went to their local church.
Sensory	John rarely feels able to join in activities but does enjoy a hand massage. John also enjoys the scent from diffusers; he finds it relaxing

It's amazing what can be achieved with the correct care.

This is just a rough guideline on how to cover each heading. Depending on the type of home you are in and also the Policies and Procedures for your company you may need to add more. You will find over time that there are things you feel are important to that person and make the Meaningful Living Plan more tailored to the person.

As with any document in the care plan, they need regular monitoring and updating. Depending on the rules where you are, these should be monitored and recorded on at least a 4 weekly basis see the document *[update sheet template]*. A sample entry is overleaf.

Any changes in the resident and the plan needs to be fully updated before a general update every 12 months.

If you are new to the role it's always best to get a nurse or team leader to review your documentation before signing it off

CARE PLAN UPDATE

NAME........Peter Jones..................................... ROOM NUMBER......7c........

DATE	UPDATE	NAME	SIGN
12/02/20	Peter enjoyed carpet bowls and wants to play again	A Smith	AS
10/03/20	Peter came along to morning worship and enjoyed singing	A Smith	AS
08/04/20	Peter enjoyed a walk in the garden and pointed out the flowers names	A Smith	AS

Plans must be updated in line with Company Policy

Chapter 5   **Good Housekeeping**

As things start to come together, the importance of good housekeeping of care plans comes into its own. Not only to meet CQC Standards but to be able to monitor the general health of the resident both physically, mentally and with activity. How often do you realise that the guy who used to shuffle along is now struggling to walk without the aid of a frame, or the lady who has gone from a few steps here and there to be full time in a wheelchair? If you don't keep your care plans updated monthly, you will have no record of when things began to change or whether there was a specific reason for that change.

How do you find the time to do this amongst facilitating all the activities you have planned?

There seems to be more and more paperwork added into our busy role: a role that many in the care sector fail to understand the importance of this. Thankfully I had great support from the start from peers and management [one activity coordinator to 40 residents] and, coming from a self-employed business background I found the paperwork fairly easy to do.

> Get to know the staff and listen to them, you'll need their support

Plan your days.

However well we plan, our days often go adrift and all for good reason. Here is a list of the average updates we need to make to keep our heads above water

ADMISSIONS

    Life Story 'This is Me'

    Photos for Care Plans

    Family Photos for a memory book and walls in the room

    The email address of NOK [next of kin]

    Introduce yourself to relatives

    If you have a social media page, you need permission from the family to allow you to use their photos. Create a document for families to sign if your company doesn't have one

WEEKLY

    Contact with residents

    Contact with Staff

    Check Activity Records are kept up to date and dispense new ones if staff are assisting

Print photos of activities for activity board and send to social media department or upload to your own home's social media pages

MONTHLY

Collect and assess activity records. Update files

Update plans in more depth when required

Activity Calendar [over time, try to get 1-2 months ahead]

Personal Reflections

Budgeting

Activity Ideas

Risk Assessment checks

Choose an Activity Person of the Month & Present Certificate

[great for motivating staff] [see templates]

6-8 WEEKS [OR AS STIPULATED]

Residents Meeting [where appropriate]

Relatives Meeting

Write up minutes & email to relatives/print for residents

QUARTERLY

Assess individual resident's activity plans

ANNUALLY

Assess all paperwork and update

Depending on your resident's ability, you may need to add your own sections to this. Also, depending on where you are and what your State legislation [if outside of the UK] requires you to complete, but your manager should be able to give you the relevant documentation for that.

What does our role *really* entail?

We are not what we seem. We are not the clown or the singer who can rattle off any song a resident requests in perfect pitch. We are, in my eyes, the lynch-pin of a well-functioning care home not just for the residents but for the staff too. We are the go-to person for sticky tape and a shoulder to lean on. We are in a metaphorical no man's land between general care staff and management: a trusted ear to one and all.

We arrange activities and often facilitate them alone

- We create activities that are person-centred to our residents
- We get to know residents as people
- We are a point of contact for families
- We organise entertainment
- We fundraise for the home
- We deal with Christmas, not just the entertainment but the parties and present buying: that's after fundraising for it of course!
- We assist at mealtimes

It's never-ending and I'm sure you can add a number more to the list. The more you get involved with the job, the more there seems to be added to your job description. The one thing that can get pushed onto activity staff from care staff is helping them out. In general, this is not a big problem especially when they are short-handed BUT don't let them come to rely on you as an extra pair of hands as you will certainly not be able to do your role to your best capability.

Set your bar when you are new to the role and remember to do it politely. 'I'm sorry but I have something to do for Mrs X but if I have time later, I'll come by' is far more acceptable than no, it's not my job. Especially when you want them to engage with activities too! A negative side effect of helping out too much is that you become behind in your job. Then what do you do? Whatever you do;

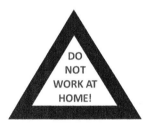

Our minds are always on the go, that comes with the territory but doing work free of charge in our own time will have a negative impact not just on your homelife but on your work life too. We need to have a healthy work/life balance. Your mind needs to rest for you to be the best you can be. Work to live not live to work!

If you cannot get every task completed in your work hours then take a look at how you manage your work time. I'm by no means implying it's your fault that you've overrun your work hours, but by assessing your daily work pattern you may see where you can make adjustments so that you can work SMART-er [SPECIFIC, MEASURABLE, ACHIEVABLE, REALISTIC, TIME BOUND] The job has its stresses that many people don't see so be careful to look after yourself and have ME time.

Be proud of what you achieve daily

Chapter 6

Working with the care staff-Motivation Awards

Many of us work alone in a care home and that is one of the toughest things to do. We just cannot do everything and it causes, as I've just said, the temptation to work from home. How can we manage? Those of you who have to have multiple activities going on every day have more than your hands full.

When I was employed it was made clear to me that I wouldn't be doing many of the activities but I would be organising them and empowering the care staff to do them. Rose-coloured glasses moment really as I thought this would be ok but little did I realise how much care staff do in their day. To be honest, it was but I fell upon the working solution, as below, by accident rather than by design.

When I went around to introduce myself to fellow staff, they were a bit nonplussed about me. The previous activity coordinator still worked in the home but she found all the paperwork too much and went on to be a regular support worker. She had done the role for about 6 months. Another carer had done the role for three months and before that, a couple of people were good but not completely person-centred. They were creating activities that they wanted to do themselves rather than for the resident.

Support the staff and ask them what activities their residents would be happy to do, get their ideas and implement them. Try not to enforce staff to do activities but empower them. Take part in these activities to show you are not shirking responsibility. The better you get on with Staff, the more likely you are to get them to facilitate activities. You are not going to get along with everyone but you can respect each other and the roles you do within the team.

Praise their actions but don't patronise, offer support and highlight little things they do that they don't already realise are a person-centred activity. By asking residents if they want tea or coffee, sitting with residents and listening to them talk about their family or where they used to live.

Empower support staff to come forward with their ideas and implement them yourself and let them take the praise. Encourage them to be involved in your planning and ask those who seem enthusiastic to assist. It's also worth bearing in mind that staff are probably doing person-centred meaningful activities without them realising it.

Giving the resident choice

Think about when you are in a restaurant and you are asked if you want mash or chips with your main meal and how much it means to you to have that choice. It's a simple thing to ask someone whether they would like custard or cream on a dessert, but it's a meaningful question to the resident. The more the staff give residents choice, the longer they will keep their independence. Don't pre-empt this decision at any time. It's all part of being person-centred: we can all change our minds! If a person has cognitive issues, give them a choice of A or B or show them pictures. Too many choices can be confusing.

Simple choices such as the following.

What they want to wear

Asking if they want tea or coffee

What they want to eat, cheese sandwich or cottage pie

Where they want to sit, at the window or the table

What they would like to do, watch TV or read a book

Converse during personal care, even play music to ease the embarrassment

Always explain what you are about to do and ask permission to do it. Even if it's as simple as moving a strand of their hair that's getting in their eyes.

Ask if they wish to join in activities or just sit and watch.

To assume that activities are just games and crafts is a big misconception. From the minute they wake up, the interaction between the resident and staff member is meaningful. That interaction of asking what the resident would like to wear today, what they would like to have breakfast and what they would like to eat and drink is a meaningful activity.

Good staff tend to do this without thinking and realising how important it is. The more our role becomes important in the home, the more I believe the title of Life Enrichment Coordinator is a better title than activity coordinator. We are all there to enrich the lives of our residents.

Short Activities

Sit and have a cup of tea and a chat

Eat your meal at the same time as you are assisting them

Hand Massage

Photo Albums

Books

Sing a Song

Give and receive a hug

Throw a ball

Bat balloons

Blow bubbles

Chat over photos

Paint nails

Jigsaw

Play music

Read the newspaper together

Peel vegetables

Listening

Skittles

Walk in the garden

Encouraging Staff Participation

Staff facilitating activities will not happen overnight. It does also depend on the staffing levels too as to how much they can do. If you have activity staff then they can facilitate.

Try these ideas

- A good way to encourage staff is to present a monthly certificate to those who work hard, show them your appreciation. *[Templates]*
- Work with the staff to help them understand how important their time is. If you have two staff with ten residents, if they spend just 15 minutes with each resident it equates to 2 ½ hours of their day
- Organise an activity rota based on their shift rota
- Randomly reward staff if they are doing well with biscuits or sweets to show your appreciation

It's finding out what works for you in your particular circumstances. Experiment and work together.

What is a big help and encouragement is to have random activities scattered around the main areas of the home. This way anyone can pick up something to do either themselves or with others. Ideas such as: -

- Rummage bags
- Quiz sheets
- Wool to sort
- Socks to pair
- Pillowcases to fold

- Veg and a peeler [peeler kept in kitchen drawer]
- Memory cards to chat from
- Newspapers and magazines
- Poetry sheets
- Balloons
- Beach ball

You will find that staff will be intrigued and start to utilise these ad hoc activities without being asked.

The other good thing about having activities scattered around the home is that it relieves some of your storage space. Some people are lucky and have storage space, an office and an activities room. Others have a broom cupboard for storage and that's it; so having activities out on the units is a great help. If you have boxes in different areas, rotate the contents weekly so there is something different.

Slowly staff will build up and be doing activities daily: but will they fill in the activity record sheets? You have the option here of filling in the sheets for them or again electing, in discussion with the management, one of the staff to ensure they are complete. This could be encompassed with the activities done by rota.

If you don't have records kept in daily record files, create a separate folder for these sheets to go into and place it in a visible place for all to acknowledge and use.

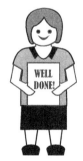

Chapter 7   Planning Meaningful Activities

'Start small, think big and you'll get there. Listen to feedback, analyse it and improve.'

Don't try and fill your activity calendar from morning to night; although I know some homes are expected to have a full calendar depending on the ability of the residents. If you are in the world of dementia, less is more.

In the beginning aim for a weekly calendar to test the waters and record the feedback of what residents enjoyed. Once you have some regular things people enjoy, build up to a monthly planner. Surprisingly, this will free up more time once you get used to doing it than a weekly calendar allows. I always felt like I was chasing my tail when doing weekly calendars!

A future step is to produce individual planners for each resident regarding room visits and personal 1:1 activity. But to do these you need to be juggling all the balls and know residents well, so I wouldn't attempt this before 6-12 months in the role. It does depend on how many residents you have and what their abilities are.

Of course, once all this planning is complete it all has to be kept up to date in line with your company's and CQC's policies and procedures. So be organised and keep things as simple as you can.

Diarize when updates need to be done and stick to it.
See what I mean about not having time to help out too.

How many activities and when to do them

Check out what supplies you will be inheriting. More than likely you will have a ton of stuff that you may never use or never think of using, but don't get rid of any of it until you know for sure that it's no use. Resident dynamics change over time so what's useful this year may not be useful next.

If you are fortunate enough to have an office, storage room and activities room, make the most of it. The only thing is that having all this wonderful space is that it keeps you away from the residents. I started my career with an 8' x 4' cupboard that was rammed to the door. The door had been left unlocked since the previous AC moved on and it was like a jumble sale. Computer time was shared with the nurses and team leaders and I often found I worked on the units with residents around me if I could get hold of a laptop.

At first, I thought this was a pain but it's a great way of absorbing the atmosphere, see how staff work and how residents behave. You have the bonus of building relationships all the time you are there, including with family members when they drop in to visit. Making them a cup of tea and having a chat is important. They can see you interacting with their loved one and you can get to know more about the family as a whole.

Listening is very important, it's amazing what you will learn. Develop the skill and you will be rewarded with information from residents and relatives as well as colleagues.

> Your work tools will be someone else's memories

Remember not to discuss information about residents with relatives unless it is your place to do so, refer them to team leaders, nurses or management. They are the ones who should be passing on relevant information. Gossiping can not only give the wrong impression; it can lead to misunderstanding.

Be tactful at all times. The funny incident of the resident doing something may come across as stupid if it's taken out of context and could horrify the relative. Always be sensitive to who you are talking to and who is listening.

Bought in entertainment

Paid for entertainment relies on you having a budget and I know a lot of people don't have anything at all. What can you get for free or cheap? What talents do the staff have or families? Cajole them to perform for the residents, maybe a karaoke afternoon or evening. How about a painting demonstration or a local choir? It's always worth approaching local schools to get visits from toddlers or a short-acting piece from secondary school. It's beneficial making these connections, especially for Christmas entertainment.

For paid entertainmen,t see if you can find out what other local homes have had. Visit and build up a list of contacts with them to get you started. Those entertainers that specialise in working in care homes often charge a lot less than those that do bars and clubs. They don't have to be the greatest singers as long as they engage with residents and the residents like them.

If you are part of a large organisation, get together via social media or an app on your phone to share ideas and offer support with others within the company if the company allows.

Always remember to book entertainers that you think the residents would like and are age-appropriate rather than what you think is nice. Be cheeky, ask the entertainer to do a free sample session or the first one at a reduced rate. I've hired several entertainers I would never pay to see personally but their capability to interact with residents and to make them happy is worth more than a singer who is pitch-perfect and doesn't connect.

Being a member of staff usually means you lose your inhibitions regarding singing in front of others so the karaoke is a great option for staff to let rip even if they are out of tune! No karaoke machine? Tune into YouTube and pick favourite tunes to belt out. At Christmas, this is great for playing carols and singing along.

Off-plan activities

So, we plan well ahead [hopefully!], we work tirelessly to deliver a varied plan for every day, but how rigidly do you have to stick to that plan?

I allow the staff to control when they deliver activities: other than those who are bought in from outside like an entertainer or the local diocese for songs of praise. They know their residents best; what time they are most receptive to activity, when they are likely to be unsettled. It's all about offering choice and not enforcing an activity onto a resident; who may not be person-centred at all.

I have a secret weapon. The Activity Box. Dotted around the communal areas are brightly coloured boxes with various activities in them such as reminiscence boxes and cards with images on to talk about, playing cards, dominoes, balloons, beach ball, poems, books to read aloud, photo books of the local area and bits of different textured material to give you an idea. This empowers the staff to have free choice over the things they do with their residents aside from the planned activities.

Spontaneous walks around the home and the grounds are popular as are staff taking the lead and having jamming sessions with the residents in a music area. Space where people donate instruments like guitars, drums, tambourines etc that can be accessed all the time.

I firmly feel that this approach is more akin to normal life than having a full day's activity schedule that residents don't want to take part in. Freedom of choice; as we would when in our own home.

Often the simplest things are the best such as chatting over a cup of coffee, chatting over a film about characters, the plot or the area it is set in. Think about what you do naturally in a day and what gives you the most pleasure. Then put yourself in a resident's shoes and think about what they may like to do and try it.

For those that are unable to go outside, bring the outdoors in. Collect seasonal leaves and branches and buds. If other residents pick some lavender, take it to the other residents to smell. You can always dry this out and make lavender bags. Buy or ask for donations of spring bulbs and pots for residents to plant up and see grow on windowsills. Don't forget the risk assessment as some bulbs are poisonous. Growing herbs that can be added to cooking or salads. Herbs are a great sensory activity as they usually have a strong scent, a great taste and some like sage leaves, an interesting texture. Allow residents to touch and sniff in their own time and go with their flow. Just because they don't engage immediately, it doesn't mean they won't next time. Learn to read body language and facial expressions to understand them. To see a resident's face light up as they scrunch autumn leaves is a delight.

If you have a resident who likes to walk a lot, see if they want to deliver the post. Someone who smooths the table cloth may like to help set the table for meals or help with the washing up. It doesn't matter if it's already been done or that you have to wash them again after, if they are keen to do it, let them. Another option is for them to help push the food trolley or the domestics cart. Someone who rarely settles into activities may enjoy helping you by putting activity packs together or filing paperwork.

There are so many things that divert us in our day to day roles that we need to just enjoy and engage with. The paperwork can wait till later, living in the now is what the resident wants.

These random engagements are often more valuable than the planned activities as it's usually the resident who starts them with you, the cook or the handyman.

Keeping it fresh

It could be said that in most circumstances repeating activities year after year is acceptable especially when your residents have dementia. But I don't believe this is the right thing to do. We ought to be continually learning and advancing with the meaningful activities we create for our residents.

People who are living with dementia change just as we do. By all means, keep a copy of last year's calendar as a base to start from [it certainly helps out with National Days and other celebrations] but don't repeat it as a whole. Be mindful of the people you are creating the calendar for.

It's inevitable that as we are looking after the elderly then they will pass on to be replaced by new residents who may be younger and have different needs. This especially covers music choice as we move from one era to the other. Be mindful of that change. 'A long way to Tipperary' will draw a blank on someone who favours Marvin Gaye.

You will soon realise how much your knowledge has increased every year so you will naturally have fresh ideas to add to the activity mix. You'll think of things that will connect better and give more stimulation. You'll think of more sensory ideas to appeal to those with advanced illnesses.

Don't be time-bound with any activity, let it flow naturally: there is no right or wrong amount of time spent doing an activity, sometimes a few minutes of engagement is enough.

When searching online, include some of the crazy days that have now been invented. Frog jumping day, dot day *[link dot day]*, doodle day *[link doodle day]* are lighthearted and can be fun.

I remember the engagement and giggles from residents as staff racing origami frogs across the floor. Priceless.

Include the odd staff activity like who can toss a pancake the most amount of times. Pre-made pancakes and an old frying pan do the trick as more often than not the pancakes end up decorating the floor! Reward the winner with a certificate and a box of chocolates. Great for team building and stress relief.

Be proud of what you achieve daily

Free or almost free

- Contact PAT dogs *[link petsastherapy]* to see if you can get a PAT dog to come into your home. They have an amazing effect on residents and are a great stress relief to staff too! Always stay with your PAT dog and handler on a visit.

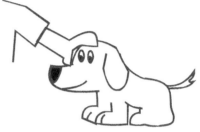

- Babies of staff. The other thing that you often see a drastic change in residents is when a baby or toddler is present.
- Contact local nurseries and schools and have young children in to play or sing. Secondary schools can do their plays or pantos for the residents. With small children, assess your residents carefully for suitability.
- Bubbles and balloons. Both give great entertainment. With bubbles, use outside to ensure no slippery residue is left on the floor.
- Baking. Use either a pre-mixed packet or mix ingredients before the session to make it easier [depending on your residents ability]. When cool they can use icing to decorate. Great fun!
- Simple things like the feel of toes in grass, sand or water.
- Use old CD's to make mobiles to hang in the trees.

- Show and tell. If residents are unable to do so, ask staff to do a ten-minute piece for the residents on their hobbies, books they read or the local environment.
- Draw around residents' hands or feet and make into a memory tree or a wreath.
- If you have cognitive residents, have a board set up with a long word written down and see how many other words they can make from it. A flip chart is perfect for this.

Group Activities

- Exercise. If you are qualified to lead then do so, but there are fitness companies around who specialise in exercise for those in a care setting.
- Mosaics. Whether with strips of paper or scrunched up tissue. Draw some guidelines on a large sheet of paper [wallpaper lining rolls are cheap and effective]. Don't forget to display it afterwards.
- Postcard share. Link up with another home and start corresponding.
- Meals out. Whether a café, restaurant or a picnic by the river. Ask staff to volunteer if you are short-handed.
- Picnic in the garden. Lovely to be out in the summer so arrange with the kitchen staff to have a picnic for a small group of residents in the home's garden.
- Indoor gardening. Planting up seeds and looking after seedlings. Ensure in your risk assessment to look into whether anyone is likely to try to eat the seedlings or soil.

- Suitcase Stories. *[Arts Uplift]* a great initiative that works well across a broad spectrum. Or create a box of memories, add some music and talk about the treasures in a case.
- Men's clubs.
- Ladies clubs.
- Travel days. Have a day in a month to explore another country. Have pictures and videos of the country and arrange with the kitchen to have food from that country on the day for lunch too.
- Shoeshine. Shoe polishing kit and box where those that can, can polish their shoes or you can do it for them.
- Reading aloud. You could have someone reading the local newspaper aloud or a quieter session with a book.
- Art and craft classes for those that are able.
- Writing classes. You could write down memories for those that can't, and arrange a tableau.
- Family anecdotes or popular sayings. You can always type these up, print, then cut in half to make a puzzle game.
- Sundown Festival. Have music at around 4 pm that residents can dance and sing along to.
- Music. Music, music, music. The number one activity for those living with dementia especially.

> Praise yourself for the knowledge you have retained and use it.

SUPPLIES

- Second-hand shops.
- Relatives and staff. Especially for raffles and fundraisers as well as creating boxes of hobbies like fishing, sewing, pipe connecting.
- Magazine images for emotions and collages.
- Flowers for flower arranging. Speak with florists and supermarkets to see if you can get the flowers they can't sell or buy some good silk ones you can use again and again.

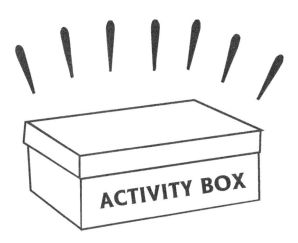

FUNDRAISING

- Book, DVD and cd sales
- Cake bake
- Weight of cake
- Sweets in a jar
- Roll a coin at a bottle
- Quiz night
- Craft sale of things made by staff
- Karaoke
- Fetes [discuss whether this is to allow the public in or just family and friends due to the vulnerability of your residents]
- Local library
- Local businesses for donations or discounts

SENSORY

- Textures, materials, paper, carpet. Textured panels on walls can make great tactile pieces when residents are walking around
- Making cakes. The feel of hands in the mix and licking the spoon!
- Garden sensory area
- Indoor gardening. Again, the feel of soil
- Reading aloud
- Fairy lights
- Scented hand creams
- Diffusers and oils
- Picture books
- Bird sounds, waves, weather videos on YouTube

Chapter 8 **Fundraising**

Budgeting for activities is a pain whether you have a large budget or none at all. All too commonly the activity staff are told to raise their own funds. Yet another skill to add to our demanding role.

Depending on your type of residents there are many things that you can do that are free or for the cost of a printout and a laminator.

Whatever size your home is there is always something you can do to raise money however small an amount it is. Cake sales to fellow staff are always a winner. Some staff love to bake and most staff love to eat! By having regular staff and relative meetings you can build up a good core group that will give you fundraising support. Don't be afraid to ask them for help, they are usually more than happy to contribute in whatever way they can.

Ensure you document and file a record of your expenditure in the Life Enrichment files on a monthly basis whether handwritten calculations or via an updated spreadsheet along with receipts.

Ideas for fundraising

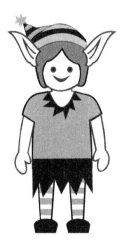

- Wear a ghastly jumper day. Ask staff for a donation for wearing that awful thing grandma bought for Christmas. You can develop this into different days across the year, like Elf day, Spotty Day or Pyjama Day.

- BBQ and fete. Charge either an admission fee or payment for food
- Summer, Spring, Autumn, Winter Fete. Either have stalls selling sweets, a tombola, second-hand books or invite local people in to sell crafts
- Quiz nights
- Music nights, get local bands involved
- Book Sale
- Cake Bake
- Craft make sessions
- Card making sessions

Ensure you publicise it well locally and with the relatives well in advance. Also, relatives are usually happy to donate for the tombola. Organise a team of people to help with the setting up: again, relatives usually come and help.

NB Always check that the company insurance covers these things and that there are food thermometers for the food and that you follow Health and Safety guidelines.

When creating activities, it is important to keep details of what the activity is and what supplies are needed. Should you move to another position either within or outside the home or be ill for a while, it is good practice to have a paper trail that others can follow.

By creating an Activity Description sheet *[see Templates]* filed in with the Life Enrichment files [see Chapter 12] you will have a record immediately on hand for yourself and others to grab quickly, and assess whether the supplies are available and whether it is suitable for the residents at that time. It's a lifesaver on mad days when you need to add in extra activities too!

Let your creative juices flow and keep events regular

ACTIVITY DESCRIPTION

NAME OF ACTIVITY ...... Balloon Tennis ....

DETAILS OF ACTIVITY

Seat residents in a circle so they are comfortable. Depending on ability you can have a net or a barrier for them to bop the balloon over or just to each other or a member of staff in the middle. If playing 1:1, be seated at a suitable distance in front of resident. Turn off the TV and play music at variable speeds to change the tempo of play

EQUIPMENT REQUIRED

Balloons

Fly Swats

Pool Noodles

GROUP.......... 1:1............. DURATION.... 15 minutes ....

EXPECTED OUTCOME

To engage residents with each other with light exercise without realising it and to have fun.

To increase interaction with staff

Chapter 9   Risk Assessments and Acceptable risk-taking

We take risks every day of our life but when we are looking after the welfare of others, we have to look at it from a different angle. We cannot cosset residents for fear of them having a fall or cutting themselves. We have to judge the risk and whether it is viable so that they can enjoy a good quality of life.

There are several good risk assessment plans on the internet but I have enclosed a simple one with a sample for you to get the feel of what you need to look at. If you have a Health and Safety Person, ask them what is necessary to include.

Should an accident occur, always report it and document it. Risk assessments should be updated annually if not sooner. Your risks may change depending on the residents you have at an activity. *[see template]*. Your company should have their generic Risk Assessment Plan for you to use.

It is possible to group risk assessments rather than do one for every single activity. For example, all craft activities could be grouped as you can look at the hazard of using pens, paints, scissors, brushes, glue etc.

There are times when you may also have to do a risk assessment for a specific individual. Usually, if they have a specific activity they do or they have a weighted blanket, although the latter should be completed by a Nurse. Keep it simple and address all the things that could go wrong.

As with any activity mentioned in this book, your own suitable risk assessment must be done before the activity taking place.

ACTIVITY RISK ASSESSMENT

ACTIVITY

Seated balloon tennis

HAZARD

Allergy to latex balloons

Trip or fall

RISK

HIGH...................... MEDIUM................... (. LOW.)......................

PRECAUTIONS IN PLACE

Ensure allergies are checked, use non latex balloons

Residents will be seated

DATE..........08/09/2020..................

Risk assessment checked by name..........Kate M........................ Review Date..08/09/21

Activity	Describe the component parts of your activity
Hazard	List things you anticipate may cause harm or things associated with your activity that have the potential to cause harm
Risk	Assess the risk as either H, M or L when concluding your assessment considering all the circumstances
Precautions	Consider what you might do to minimise/negate the risks
In place	Will the precautionary measures be in place at the time of the activity
Review Date	When would it be reasonable to review your assessment
Reviewer	Name of the person responsible for completing the risk assessment

Chapter 10   Unit Meetings/Group Meetings

Staff meetings are important and should take place regularly; every 4-6 weeks. This is a good time to keep staff updated on things going on in the home, to praise the positives, to promote future events and ask for assistance and build your relationship with them. It's also an important time for staff to feel comfortable in airing matters they want to discuss that doesn't need a one to one meeting. It's important if this happens that you listen and take their concerns and ideas seriously. Don't forget night staff too, try to schedule a meeting so that they can attend.

Ensure you advertise meetings well in advance and ask if anyone wants to discuss anything specific. Twilight activities are important for those who don't settle well, so ensure night staff are aware of the Activity Boxes and tell them how they can contact you for anything special they may need to engage fully with a resident.

Residents' and Relatives meetings

It is good practice and policy that you hold residents' meetings. This is practical for those that are cognitive but can be quite difficult with those who are bedridden or have mid/late stage dementia.

 The purpose of these meetings is to find out from the residents what they want you to achieve for them within the home. Good for feedback for you to assess your activities and see what new things you can bring in.

It is helpful if you can have the odd support worker present too who can assist if residents need help and also, they can see what you do in your role and hopefully come onside to facilitate activities.

Meetings give residents the chance to air any grievances they may have and helps both you and them to build a solid relationship.

Relatives meetings are a way to update families of what is going on in the home and what ideas you are developing. Building up a good relationship with relatives can give you a whole new section of volunteers, ideas and donations. They can be a great support to any venture that you are trying to get moving, and of course they have an inside track on residents. You can also find out what they would like to discuss during meetings. We are here to support families as well as their loved ones.

Pitfalls

You are always going to get some people in a meeting who either try to dominate or divert away from the agenda. You have to be firm. Any other business can come in at the end but make a point of saying at the beginning that personal issues are not to be discussed. If anyone wants to raise personal issues they can do so afterwards and you will signpost them in the right direction.

Minutes need to be taken and stored appropriately as well as distributed to attendees and acted upon a set time scale. If you can have a member of management or a peer to write minutes, that allows you to concentrate on controlling the meeting. A meeting should last in the region of 1 hour. Be prepared to move the meeting on if things are dragging.

There is both an Agenda and a Minutes template in the Templates chapter where I have filled in small details for you to work from.

At the end of the Template chapter is a link to obtain the spreadsheets and templates as a download via email so that you can adapt them to suit your home.

To give your best, you must be at your best

Chapter 11   **Newsletter**

Communication is a big part of our role and newsletters allow us to communicate with everyone from staff to residents and families. Newsletters are a great way to pass on information, highlight events coming up and show pictures of happy smiling residents. Staff also enjoy featuring in the newsletters, especially if they have won an award, completed a charity walk or run or developed an idea for within the home.

Newsletters take time to collate so don't commit yourself to do them too frequently unless you have time to. Templates can be found on the internet, if you can't find anything suitable, create a news sheet. Don't do too many pages to start with, add slowly as you balance your working day.

Good things to add to the newsletter are staff recipes, jokes and short stories, even a profile of a staff member answering questions that you wouldn't normally know the answer to. One of our staff found out she has Royal blood: even if it is many times removed from the mainline!

Newsletters are a great way of showing families 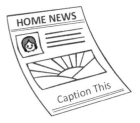 what residents have been doing in the home. You can print these off for staff to read aloud, visiting relatives to take away or email them. Use the Newsletter to appeal for donations for fetes, assistance in planting bulbs in the garden, or help in organising the Christmas Party.

> Make it feel like home for residents and family

Chapter 12 **Life Enrichment Files**

We have all seen Care Plan folders that are bulging at the seams; one day they break apart and end up in an ungainly heap on the floor. So let's separate the <u>non-essential</u> activity paperwork for our filing system so that we can access it readily rather than trawling through hefty Care Plans. It is worth compiling a separate set of files that sit alongside the Care Plans to evidence your role and the participation of the residents.

This is going to vary depending on where you are and the Policies and Procedures of your company, so add to the files what you need. This is where you would link the resident's information to the Meaningful Living Plan that is in their main care plan. All the information here is important but more to you than the nurses. It's nice to have all your residents' information together so that you can refer to it at a moment's notice.

File 1   Residents 'This is Me', Permission to use photographs on Social Media and Activity Record Sheets. Record Sheets can mount up so archive them every three to six months*.

     *Ask admin what the procedure is for this and comply

     We need to be mindful to comply with GDPR at all times.
     [General Data Protection Regulation]

File 2   Entertainers Details [including cost, when used and likes and dislikes], Risk Assessments and Budgeting and Activity Description.

File 3   Meeting Minutes, Newsletters, Feedback from Relatives and Residents, Feedback Forms

Ensure all staff are aware of these files so that they can use them as a reference. These files can then be accessed by professionals who come in and needs to evaluate a resident and their inclusion in activities without having to trawl through medical notes. At all times, files should be kept in a secure location where they are unavailable to anyone not specified to access them.

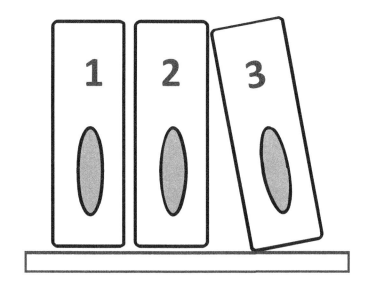

Chapter 13   Nutrition and hydration

Nutrition and hydration can be fun as well as necessary

All jobs within a care setting are important to you, it could be said that that you can become the elastic between departments as well as a shoulder to lean on and a negotiator. It all depends on you and the relationships you build up with those around you.

Ensure you form a good relationship with the kitchen staff. You'll lean on them for birthday cakes, party food, dietary advice, event catering, celebration days, whacky ideas and all sorts.

Fish and chip Friday is a great example. Help wrap the food in greaseproof and newspaper for residents to eat from. Have condiments to add and you have a joyful sensory lunch. Again, teamwork is important and the kitchen can be a fountain of knowledge.

A balanced diet is very important in a care home and this should be addressed by the dietary department/kitchen. What we can do is increase hydration when it is hot by way of having extra fluids and fruits as part of an activity.

Fruit tasting is a great option as well as having a mocktail session with new flavours. Dress these up with cocktail stirrers and umbrellas and a small amount of fresh fruit. Every little helps, and it is also a way of working with the support workers to builds good working relationships. It's worth keeping a separate list of allergies and intolerances just in case someone is allergic to strawberries or dairy products. Also, whether they need thickener in liquids or not. ***Never give anyone food or fluids unless you are aware of their requirements and remember to report back to support staff who*** *are keeping the daily notes.* In the winter, do warm drinks like cocoa or as a treat, chocolate and churros.

In the warmer months, cocktail parties serving mocktails and chunks of fruit are a great winner for everyone. Remember to cut fruit small enough so that it doesn't become a choke hazard.

You can turn this into an extra activity by asking residents to identify the ingredients in the mocktail or what the fruit is. Often this will bring out memories such as 'when I was little we used to climb into the farmers field and help ourselves to strawberries'. It's important we allow residents to tell these stories and discuss it with them.

Access and control your budget. **DO NOT** spend your own money

Chapter 14   **Sensory Therapy**

For those of us that are working with those living with mid to late-stage dementia, devising meaningful activities can often be difficult and stressful. Crafts and games are often too difficult for them to either take part in or for their brain to cope with. So how can we connect with these residents?

We need to approach them utilising the five senses of touch, smell, sight, sound and taste. Not a new concept but an important one. Joyce Simard cumulated her knowledge to bring us the Namaste way of Care *[ref Joyce Simard]* and we have found that this is a great therapy to use regularly with residents. It does not need to cost a lot to set it up, just a little ingenuity.

With the Namaste way of care, it is useful for those not just in the later stages of their dementia journey but for those that don't want to join in group activities or who have additional illnesses to dementia. The chance for these residents to have some dedicated 1:1 care regularly has an amazing impact on their quality of life and mood. The University of Worcester ADS *[ref Worcester University]* have trialled Namaste Care for the last few years and found it a worthwhile therapy to offer. You can achieve the Namaste experience with very little outlay.

Building a Namaste/sensory room is not as ominous as it sounds. If you are fortunate enough to have a spare room with enough space to fit in a couple of chairs with arms, then you could convert it. Otherwise, you could section off an area of a lounge, conservatory or activity space. If we take each sense in turn, it will give you some idea of how it can be achieved with very little outlay.

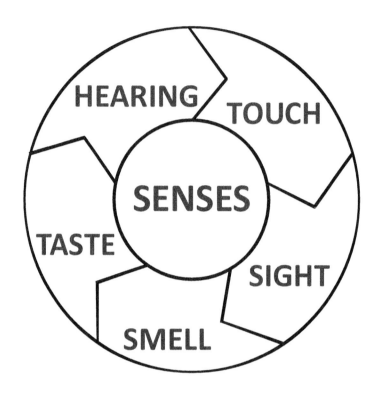

Touch   Textured materials, water, creams, teddy bears.
        Hand and foot massage with scented lotions [be
        mindful of allergies], twiddle muffs and blankets.
        With massage be aware of residents with arthritis.
        Never try to straighten their fingers out. *Close your
        eyes and imagine what around you has texture.*

Smell   Sweet peas, herbs, aromatherapy oils in a bottle [only
        put oil on a small piece of cotton wool in a suitable

container, NEVER on the skin], chocolate. Again, think with your eyes shut.

Sight	Not everyone has good eyesight, but having a TV in the area linked to the internet opens up your options for dedicated viewing of relaxing videos on YouTube of beautiful scenery, the sea, birds, favourite music. Have at hand photos to talk about that are enlarged so the resident can see them. Fairy lights that change colour [avoid fast-paced change sequence as this could cause a fit] around the room or ones that can be handled. Anything the resident will find relaxing.
Sound	Music is a lifesaver. I've never known a resident not like to listen to their favourite music and tap their fingers or feet, sing or smile. Don't have it too loud or it may agitate the residents involved. Favourite music, bird song, reading aloud, poetry, talking one to one.
Taste	Mocktails, seasonal fruits, sharp and sweet flavours. Try to include different textures and sweet and savoury. Be aware of any allergies that residents may have. As a group activity in a daily setting, have a fish and chip day. Work with the kitchen on this and deliver the fish and chips to residents wrapped in greaseproof then newspaper. The traditional English way. Engage staff so that they deliver the packages to residents for them to open themselves and to eat directly from the paper-like we all do when visiting a chip shop.

Have on hand salt and vinegar to enhance this sensory time. If you are able, add the options of curry sauce, gravy and mushy peas.
You will find that for the majority, the appetite increases and people who normally avoid plated fish and chips will eat heartily.

Refer to the Meaningful Living Plan to see what are the residents favourite flavours, smells and hobbies.

Record your session on the Interaction Record Sheet *[see templates]*and highlight anything that produced an impact on the resident be it positive or negative. The Sensory Room has lots of other positive uses. Here are a few.

- The Sensory Room can also be a great place to take residents that are escalating in their mood. If you can see the signs that they will become agitated, ask if they would like to go there and listen to some favourite music.
- Space for couples to spend time together rather than the communal lounge or the resident's room. Monitor this in accordance with the resident's care plan and company policy.
- An area for a staff member to go if they are feeling stressed after an altercation with a resident or the passing of a favourite resident.

You will need to lead by example to ensure staff take residents to this space and teach them massage techniques and explain what it is all about. Also, highlight that they get one to one contact with residents in a relaxed unhurried atmosphere.

This is a basic set up for a sensory room or area, you can add more yourself as you get the feel for it and the budget allows. You can purchase specific elements to make up a sensory room from specialist suppliers so if you can get funding from management or fundraise, go for it.

- This sensory time must be calm and relaxed
- Don't have too many residents in the area at once
- Start with residents who don't join in much or who get little interaction or visitors
- Residents may be hesitant at first but persevere. Even if it is just going in there to enjoy a cup of tea and a biscuit with you
- Some residents will never use the sensory area and that's OK
- Never leave a resident in the sensory area unattended
- Encourage families to engage with you and their resident by giving hand massages or quality together time when you haven't got a group in place
- Agitated family visitor? Take them into the sensory area to relax
- Always keep lighting low and slowly increase light and sound in preparation to leave the session
- How long should a session last? That depends on the residents involved. If someone wants to leave after 15 minutes allow them to do so and quietly escort them so as not to disturb others
- Staffing. Ideally, a session should be on a 1:1 or 1:2 basis so that the resident gets undivided attention from you. As you are putting the area in place, talk with staff and pick the keenest ones to begin the sensory journey with residents. A taster session with staff so they get the feel of it is

invaluable. The sensory session is relaxing for staff too but can be tiring if it goes on for an hour or more, so allow them a 5-minute break after residents have finished a session

- Sensory sessions should be a daily occurrence for all residents but it can be impossible to achieve this with the limited staff available. Trials have shown that residents who use the sensory area are frequently calmer and more responsive than when they didn't have the sessions in place
- Always ensure the area is left clean and tidy ready for the next group
- Do not wear gloves when giving a massage. This comes across more like personal care and not a sensory experience
- Keep records so that you can evaluate the improvement or not of a resident who goes to sessions. Staff can complete these whilst the lights are going up and the resident listens to a favourite piece of music at the end

Chapter 15　　**Personal Reflection**

Life passes us by at an alarming rate especially when we are in a new role. We are constantly learning and achieving; our heads are full of information and we fail to realise how much we have achieved.

Keep a notebook with you at all times. Not only to jot down requests from residents and families but also to write down the bare bones of an idea and things you need to address.

I have always found it an advantage to review my performance monthly to see where my knowledge gaps are, where I am excelling and, whether I am reaching the targets I've set myself. [See templates]. I find it interesting to look back on these when I am due supervision and also if I am having a low point; feeling frustrated. We are always quick to knock ourselves but not quick enough to praise ourselves for what we achieve and believe me, we achieve a lot!

"SB smiled at me today and made eye contact"

"RS relaxed in the chair and enjoyed a hand massage"

"TW said she wanted to go into the garden to pick flowers"

"DR sang in the church service"

I don't need to expand on these because you all know how important these seemingly little things are and nine times out of ten, they bring a lump to our throat and a tear to our eye.

Never underestimate how important you are to the lives of these people.

Whether it is during peer reviews or at any other time we are always going to get someone who disagrees with the way we do things. Management may disagree with an activity; families may think something you are having great success with is childish. How do we respond?

It is very easy to defend ourselves immediately but is that the best course of action? Probably not. The reason we react is that our feelings have been hurt and we want to defend ourselves. It is better to listen than react and think about what that person is saying to you and why.

Try to find out why people disagree with an activity. A family member may see something as childish because they are remembering that person when they were fit and able. Seeing them do something simple is an indicator that that person will never be the same again. The relative may feel responsible for the resident's state of health even though they can do nothing about it. We blame ourselves for things we truly cannot control.

Try to understand things from their perspective. Of course, if you have a relative who is constantly criticising you and what you do, speak with your manager to discuss the best way of handling the situation; your manager may know more than you do about the circumstances and can advise you accordingly and also have a chat with the family to see what their issues are regarding. You may just be bearing the brunt of their anxiety.

If management criticises you, they will usually do it during peer review and it will be explained why this has come to their attention. They will have thought it through before discussing it so listen and take note of their concerns. If you go away thinking you have been hard done by, write down why you feel that way and meet with the manager again to discuss your feelings and how things can be improved. None of us are perfect.

Chapter 16   **Passing your Inspection**

The million-dollar question for all of us in care is how do we do our best to ensure we get through with a clean sheet and get high grades for our CQC. I can only go on the UK as is my experience, which I have to say was a pleasant one! They were in and out within a day but continued to ask questions after their visit before giving the home I worked in 4 outstanding and 1 good. Top 3% in the country!

From the perspective of the Activity role, I would anticipate it is all very similar in that we need to document everything in a clear way that not only conforms to our company's Policies and Procedures but also conforms to the examining body's criteria.

Whatever area you are in, access the criteria from the examining board of your area, create yourself a spreadsheet and check yourself off against it. There is also the option that the company may have the previous year's checklist and you can work against that. In the UK, this is where the Life Enrichment Files come in very useful as supporting evidence.

Check other homes that are similar to yours online at the *CQC [see CQC]* and see what their report is like, measure your own home against that report and see where you have areas that you feel can be improved upon. Read through some outstanding reports and aim towards achieving the same standards. Even in outstanding homes, there is always room for improvement.

The day of your inspection arrives. Depending on previous inspections and size etc of your home, the CQC will visit for one or two days, sometimes more. DON'T PANIC! Go about your day to day routine and offer them as much help as they request. Excuse yourself if you need to proceed with an activity that is scheduled and invite them along. They will want to see your documentation for each resident and want to know how you came to the conclusion about the activities that you are offering and why they are suitable. If you have all your documentation in separate files to the care plan, it's a much easier process.

Always ensure that the necessary files are in the care plan so that they can be referenced across from one to the other. The Life Enrichment Files need to be easily accessible to the staff but, like care plans, not easily available to anyone else or you will violate GDPR. As previously mentioned, they need to be updated every three to four weeks so that all information is current and suitable for the resident.

Think about how you answer the inspectors; they know you are likely to be nervous but they are not trying to deliberately catch you out. We are a special breed and they know how much other areas rely on our role in the care home. If you don't understand a question, ask them to rephrase it.

The more relaxed you are the more relaxed the staff around you will be. Lead by example and if you have time, encourage staff to relax and be positive.

We are not perfect. But when CQC come in, we can go into a flap about everything.

Mentally step back and look around you to ensure as many things are in place as you'd like them to be. Mentally prepare to tell the CQC about all the little things you have in place that they may not be able to see on their walk around the home. About the poetry-reading you do for Doris who is bed-bound, the garden walk and naming of plants with Joe, the ice cream van that visits where staff bring residents out to queue for ice cream.

When they have finished chatting to you, they may come back again if they think or see something they'd like answered.

When you have relaxed, have a short break and write down some notes on the things they asked you so that you can report back to your manager on what you were asked.

If you are doing your job well, you will have no problems with the inspection. How well you pass will depend on how the inspectors think you and the whole team at the home are doing. We can only do what we can do. Most homes just have one Activities person which means we are running around all the time and they understand that. If you are fortunate to have assistants, ensure they are up to speed with documentation as well as the delivery of activities.

Good Luck!

If the inspector says something to you that you think can be rectified on the spot, report to your manager immediately so that it can be dealt with

Chapter 17   **LGBT+**

Society is more open about a person's gender and lifestyle choices than it has ever been before with people also being able to identify as gender-neutral or gender fluid. Being rehoused into a care setting can be quite upsetting to them and the acceptance of those around them when they have lived a private life in their community.

There are more and more LGBT+ residents than ever before and we have to learn to adjust to their needs as much as anyone else's. We have to be aware that there may be discrimination amongst staff and fellow residents.

We cannot give blanket rules on this as each person and their needs are different. We need to be aware though that their settling in period and their needs may be slightly different to others and respect their rights and privacy as you would anyone else.

N.B. if you are working with dementia, this can throw up the added complication with transgender that when the person is regressing to their past life, they may wish to be called a different name of the other gender. It's a case of go with the flow and do your best to accommodate their needs the same as anyone else.

> We are all human

Chapter 18   Making new residents feel at home

It's distressing for anyone coming into a home whether it's for the first time or whether they are changing homes. It is important to make them feel welcome.

- Have a card waiting for them with some flowers or a small gift
- Ensure you meet them as soon as possible to start building up a relationship
- Meet the family and get them to sign a form to allow you to use their image for social media [if they wish to]
- Give the family a 'This is Me' booklet to fill in and return
- Find out what you can about the new resident from families; sometimes you may not see them again
- Introduce new residents to other residents and make them feel at home
- Add their name to their door
- Create a memory box for outside their door from photos and precious things
- Find out what their previous professions and hobbies were

Give them time to settle in before you do a personal evaluation. They may feel afraid, angry, upset, so reassure them as much as you can.

Chapter 19   **Dementia**

One in three of us will develop dementia, it's a sobering thought. With a large proportion of care and nursing home residents having dementia, it is important that we have some understanding of the dementias and how it affects those living with it.

The more common dementias are: -

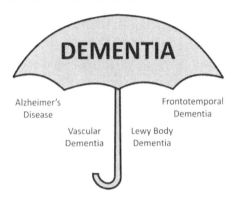

Young Onset is becoming more common too.

A valuable resource is the Alzheimer's Society, *[Alzheimers]* Here you can read the typical symptoms of the above dementias and also about the less common ones.

What is most important to those of us working with those living with dementia is to understand how they react and behave with the disease and how we try to help them live the best life possible. There is no handbook for this, what works for one person may not necessarily work for another. But by delivering person-centred care and activities we can help residents live a good quality of life.

Don't assume that someone aggressive will always be aggressive. We need to look into why they are aggressive. Are they bored, in pain or feeling lonely? Can we increase contact with this resident and by working on The Meaningful Living Plan find a meaningful activity that would stimulate them and in doing so decrease their aggression?

Someone comes in who is bedbound for no medical reason, it is the resident's choice to remain in bed. You discover by chatting to them that they were bored in the last home and no one ever paid her any attention so she took to her room and then got depressed and stayed in bed. With increased chats and smiles, this lady wants to sit in the chair by the window and slowly but surely, she wants to see the rest of the home.

A Young Onset Dementia resident loses his temper and starts shouting and throwing things and he needs personal care. Personal care is difficult as the resident is still angry, but why? Because of the type of dementia he has, he is aware that he was unable to get to the bathroom before he had an accident. He's angry at himself and not at staff. Playing music can aid in calming him enough to receive personal care. By pre-empting his bathroom habits some of this aggression can be eliminated.

As those with dementia do not calm down very quickly, asking the resident if they would like to go and sit in the quiet and listen to some of their favourite music can help deviate their mind from the incident. This is also where the sensory room can come in very useful.

Keeping those with dementia as active as possible not only gives them a better quality of life but is also beneficial to the staff who are delivering care.

"I want to go home"

A sentence often heard in a dementia home from a large portion of residents. But where is home? Spend a moment thinking about where you would call home and write down a few ideas below.

I can almost guarantee that you have named a house you live in, your parent's home, a town or country. But this is not always the answer for someone with dementia. Home is more often a feeling. A feeling of comfort, happiness, security at a point in their life where they were happy. This could mean they are missing something in their life currently. A gap we try to unravel and see how we can fill it. Asking if they would like to bake cakes, help lay the table or wash up can be a simple solution.

Working in the dementia field is challenging and draining at times. You are like a detective trying to find clues in what people say even when it makes no sense to you, you have conversations about things you never knew existed, you learn to understand people's vocal sounds to know if they are happy, sad or in pain. It's hard work but those smiles I mentioned earlier are truly rewarding.

I could write a whole book on dementia but for now, please delve into the links at the rear if you wish to study more on dementia. There are free and paid-for courses that you can take to improve your CPD plus general information to help in your work.

Don't assume the resident asleep in the chair is resting, they may be bored with nothing to do or listening to conversations around them.

Chapter 20   **Volunteers and Students**

Volunteers can be a blessing especially if you have no assistants, but they need to have the right approach to your specific residents to make it work. But how do we find volunteers?

The church near the home may have some members who would like to come in once a week or once a month to chat with residents over a cup of tea. Or they could do some woodworking with the men, flower arranging with the ladies; or vica versa. Maybe they could do some baking too.

Having that extra pair of hands for a few hours here and there not only take the pressure off you, but could also provide a fresh face that residents look forward to seeing. It's the little things that can make a big difference. Staff or visitors may also know someone who would happily come in; just ask!

Never leave volunteers alone with residents until they feel comfortable to do so and only if your company policy allows or they have a suitable DBS*. Give them time to adjust to their surroundings and get to know a few of the residents.

It is worth offering volunteers some training about the behaviours of people in your home in general terms and how to safeguard themselves and the residents. This may take extra time from your day but it reaps its rewards as volunteers will feel more confident in the environment.

Check with your manager to see if DBS checks are necessary.

Students are a common feature in care homes. They are usually at college studying Health and Social Care and have to do so many hours a year placement as part of their course.

Approach your manager and then the local college to see if you can offer a placement for one or two days a week. Hopefully, you will get a willing candidate who can assist you in facilitating meaningful activities for the residents. They become especially helpful at busy periods like Christmas when there are parties to organise, presents to shop for and wrap.

The student gets a taste of what it's like to work in the environment before they make a career choice at the end of their course. Again, they will need a DBS check but the college normally sorts this.

Spend time with students to make them comfortable in the environment. Remember they are young and may well have not ever visited a care or nursing home so will be unfamiliar with not only how the place works but the behaviours of residents too.

The students will need ongoing support from you and the team. If you can buddy them up with a member of staff for a while, they will learn more that way too.

Remember they are learning Health and Social Care so don't just give them menial jobs to do, structure their day with that in mind. Most will always enjoy being part of activities and they are a much-needed pair of hands at Christmas when you have so much to do.

Chapter 21   **Training & Self-Management**

Currently, in the UK, there are no qualifications required for you to become an Activities Coordinator/ Life Enrichment Coordinator which is unlike the USA. But there are courses you can take to improve your CPD and hopefully improve your job prospects. Most of these courses are available online or, if you are lucky, your company itself will put you in for the NAPA QCF in Supporting Activity in Social Care [level 2] or Activity Provision in Social Care [level 3] *[see links].* Take a look at the website to see more in-depth details.

Online, there are also free courses you can do via Future Learn or MOOT *[see links].*

Additional training will always be a positive addition to your CV.

One of the things you will need to work on at all times is personal time management. Yes, you can receive training for this but only you know what your role entails with the complexity of the residents in your home. You won't always get it right and at times you'll be chasing your tail but try to manage your time efficiently.

Let's say you are working full time and 8-hour days with a 30-minute lunch break. Write down what you HAVE to do during a month as I've previously listed. Calculate how long on average it takes you to resource, collate and write up the monthly calendar. 'Add in the activities you have brought in that take place at a particular time/day. Add anything else that is cast in stone. When you have this, you can balance yourself with the activities you are doing. Don't cram this plan as you know that there will be random things cropping up that will take your time, such as; *'you go to reception to put up next month's calendar, Joyce is sitting looking out of the window. She sees you and smiles and calls you over. You pull up a chair and chat with Joyce about the people walking past and the flowers she can see. An hour later and Joyce wants a snooze so you escort her to her room where she asks to go'.* It doesn't matter that you have been delayed from finishing a project because you have just been part of something pleasurable for Joyce.

Monday to-do list
Start working on next month's calendar for approx. 2 hours
Call Joyce's daughter about a hair cut
Request finances for activity art supplies

The activity calendar shows

Monday Activities
Am   Reading aloud from 10-11
Talk to Lottie whilst she eats her lunch
Pm   Songs of Praise

- You have to learn to manage your time to juggle all these things. If you haven't done it before, pre-prepare a selection of books for residents to choose what you read from.
- Have your finance request ready and agree on a suitable time with Admin to gain the funds.
- Find the number for Joyce's daughter

- Get the room ready for Songs of Praise and remind staff that it is taking place and you need residents there by a specific time
- Organise the seating in the service so everyone can see and be seen, that those who like to walk around are free to do so and those that may wish to leave early have a clear path.
- Ensure your placement of chairs and residents leaves suitable access for exiting the building should the alarm go off
- Think about the personalities coming into the room and where they are seated to get the best experience.

What looks like a few simple things to some is quite in-depth when you analyse it. I can guess that planning the calendar may end up being passed to another day! But that doesn't matter as long as you allow yourself enough time to get on with it through the month.

Chapter 22 **Birthdays**

Always, always, always, have an up to date birthday list of your residents. Ensure Management and the kitchen have a copy too.

But what should we do for birthdays? That's going to depend on the budget available and your manager's thoughts too.

Do you have a monthly party to celebrate all birthdays that month?

Do you give cards and presents?

Do you bake a cake and erect banners?

Will the kitchen make birthday cakes or will you buy them?

It's these things that need looking at and, depending on what you decide, have birthday packs ready for each resident with banners, balloons and cards ready in advance. Of course, the balloons then come in handy for a quick game of Balloon Tennis!

Chapter 23   **What is an Activity?**

Jot a few things down here as to what you think an activity is.

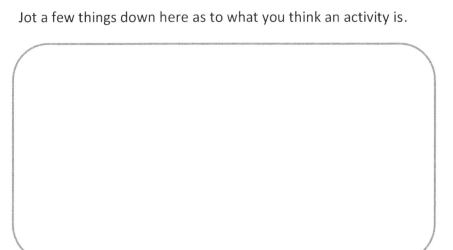

We all have different views on what constitutes an activity depending on our residents. No activity is right or wrong as long as residents are getting something meaningful from it.

As I said originally, I won't cover pages and pages of activities as there are so many resources available on the internet for free that we can all access. Just ensure that the activities you put on your calendar are suitable for your residents, meaningful to them and that you don't set them up to fail by giving them an activity that is too difficult for them to understand or take part in.

Your company could also subscribe to one of the many companies that provide online resources directly to you. They have ideas for activities, printouts ready to use, helpful hints themed days and some can even do your monthly calendar for you. Are they worth it? That is for you to decide.

Memory Cards.

I created memory cards for many reasons. They are an A4 sheet of paper or card with a photograph on such as a 1960's wedding. On the reverse are a set of questions to help the staff member use the card within a 1:1 or group setting such as

- Where did you get married? [please be sure the resident has been married before asking that one]
- How many people were at your wedding?
- What was it like?
- Were you ever a Best Man or Bridesmaid?

These few simple questions help get a conversation started. They are good for anyone visiting too. Sometimes a conversation can be a bit stilted, we all get tongue-tied at times so having a starting point for a visitor is helpful to them. Do a whole range covering holidays, cars, clothes, school, sports and leave them in Activity boxes to be used again and again.

Do you have residents sitting at the dining table looking bored whilst others are assisted to their seats? Print off some bright coloured images of fruits, vegetables, animals that you can engage these residents with whilst everyone is getting seated and the meal is served.

- Discuss what fruits and vegetables they like
- Did they have a pet?
- How many oranges can you see?
- Point and ask to name a vegetable as you have forgotten

Both of these ideas are cost-effective and once you laminate them, they can last for months.

Children

There is something special about seeing an elderly person respond to the presence of young children. Liaise with a local nursery about visiting to allow the children to just play in the middle of the room whilst residents watch on, or Brownies or Cubs. Ensure you have a Risk Assessment in place and enough staff on hand to deal with any issues should they occur. The nursery will bring enough staff to cover their children. This can take a while to get organised as it has to be discussed with the children's parents but it is worthwhile, especially for those who never get to see their grandchildren.

Music

Music never fails. Whether it's live singing from a choir or playing old records. Every type of music has a positive effect. There are a lot of singers and musicians who specialise in visiting care homes. Hold on to the good ones as they are worth their weight in gold. You can also get residents playing music even if you don't have instruments: make your own! Plastic milk bottles with some sand or stones in to shake [just glue them shut], scrunchy paper makes a great sound, a plastic tub [catering size from the kitchen] or an empty sweet tub make great drums.

Reminiscence Therapy

Think of something you did for a holiday as a child, what emotions does the memory bring back?

We all reminisce whatever age we are. Harking back to the days when things were cheaper, fashion trends, our favourite chocolate. How do we use reminiscence with residents?

There is the Suitcase Stories Scheme *[see link]* that will come to your home with a musician and historical objects or you can create your reminiscence activities in the home.

- Create boxes of themed items
  By the Sea; a stick of rock, sand, the sound of seagulls, comics, knotted hankie
- Wedding; confetti, place-cards, horseshoe, wedding cards, material, invitations
- Sports; football, rugby ball, football programme, boots, whistle, yellow card, side-line flags
- Hobbies; knitting, sewing, crochet, handmade toys, patterns

Outside the resident's room, you can have memory boxes with their precious photos in, trinkets that mean a lot to them, a bottle of special scent or aftershave.

You can also book period singers to enter your home from Elvis to Madonna!

Getting out and about.

On a beautiful summers day there is nothing nicer than being out in the sun, so with a fellow member of staff take a small group out for a walk.

- Don't forget sun cream and sunhats
- Ensure medication is taken and all paperwork needed is with you such as DNR's
- Ensure wheelchairs are sound and lap belts are done up

- Check out the walk before you take residents out. What may be easy for you and me could be a trip hazard or be impossible to negotiate in a wheelchair
- Take money for ice creams!
- Don't forget to do a risk assessment

If you are in an area you can't walk from safely, call the local ice cream van company and ask them to visit. They will usually be happy to do so for a small cost. It is hard work getting all residents out to the van to get ice cream [please don't spoil their enjoyment by getting it for them unless they are unable], but seeing the joy on their faces as they hold that cone is worthwhile.

Minibus

Not everyone is lucky enough to have a minibus and if your home has one you may be asked to be its driver. A minibus opens up a whole other world of activity. Trips out into the countryside or the theatre.

Ensure you know how many passengers able-bodied and wheelchairs it can hold. Know your residents and seat them on the minibus to suit their possible behaviours and patience whilst everyone gets on.

Don't forget to include support staff in these numbers too as you will need to have help. Plan ahead and ensure there are staff available for the trip and take along everything your residents are likely to need; even if it is just a trip to the supermarket 10 minutes away.

Impromptu activities

I prefer to call this 'living in the moment'. This is something that occurs totally off the cuff and unplanned and it often brings the best rewards. It can come in various ways from sitting helping Beryl with her sewing, George assisting the Maintenance Man as he fixes a shelf or a sing-song with a group of residents. The list is endless and unplanned. Enjoy that moment as much as the resident does.

Calendar

Working on the months calendar is the bane of our lives in some ways. It takes us away from the residents we do our job for but is necessary so that we are well planned. There is no right or wrong way to do a calendar. I prefer to keep a calendar quite loose as working in the world of dementia, things can change in the blink of an eye.

- Ensure the calendar is clear and concise with allotted times and locations when necessary.
- Print and put on all notice boards and also remind staff when they are required to assist in residents moving to another location for the activity.
- If you are giving calendars to residents, ensure the print is of a size that they can read easily. In this instance, it may be easier to print it out week by week.
- Keep it varied and interesting

Christmas

Christmas is the biggie for everyone in care. It's teamwork with turbo power! I always start planning Christmas in September/ October, crazy but necessary.

- Start asking for donations for raffle prizes [if you have very little storage space you get creative about where to store them!]
- Budgeting. If you don't have a budget you need to fundraise
- Start writing the residents Christmas cards; it's tiring
- Buy the essentials like rolls of wrapping paper, tags and sticky tape
- Liaise with the kitchen about Christmas dinner and the timing
- Don't forget Santa!!
- Will you choose a theme for the home? I let staff decide on a theme for different areas and then in October/November supply them with materials. And yes, this was on the calendar as an activity too!
- Entertainment. Book earlier than September if you can as entertainers get booked solid
- Carol service. Hold this separately in the home or if you are able, go to the local church. Have a chat with the vicar. If you have to use the minibus to get there, good luck, it takes hours to get residents on, strapped in and off again; then the reverse procedure. But once again, it is truly worth the effort
- Organise a Christmas Committee made up of staff and relatives to help you. It's hard work doing it alone
- Christmas tree[s]. Call around and see who will donate you one or two

- Table decorations. An easy make is to trim off excess Christmas tree branches and glue them together flat, add some baubles and glitter and hey presto
- If you are not covered in glitter from November to Christmas, can you tell me your secret?

Chapter 24   **End of Life**

It's a sad fact that we all have to face but we will lose residents during our time in a home and it is upsetting to all the staff. But our job is to ensure that the resident has the best quality journey.

With the rare odd exception, most residents will become ill and take to their bed so how do we deal with this situation? What we don't do is just ignore them, they have changed and we need to change with them.

- Relaxing music
- Reading poetry aloud or their favourite book
- Taking to them
- Take time to listen to what they have to say
- Allow family private time and have tissues and bottled water available or make them tea/coffee when they visit
- Use of the sensory area. If you can get the resident along to the sensory area, they may benefit from the hand massages or lights. If not, take the therapies to them

Do your best, it's not easy. There's no reason to be ashamed of shedding tears at the passing of someone you have grown fond of.

Chapter 25   **Lockdown**

It can be the most testing time of all when there is an epidemic in the home. Germs and diseases can spread quickly from one area to another so it may mean that at some point your home or parts of it go into lockdown. This means that some or all of your residents are confined to their rooms for their health and safety. But like the support workers, our role continues.

It can be difficult for residents who are well to understand why they are confined to their room, often an explanation is met with blank looks and even anger.

At this time the calendar goes out the window as we try to keep residents occupied.

- Management will make the decision and we all follow Policies and Procedures.
- Health and Safety is a priority. Disinfecting supplies we give out and ensuring we are gloved and masked in between each room visit.
- Creativity comes to the fore in utilising anything we have that the resident can enjoy doing

By following the rules, viruses rarely last longer than a week or two. Just stay safe and report anything you see that is not normal for that resident.

Chapter 26 **Templates**

Interaction Record Sheet

Update Sheet- Care Plan

Meaningful Living Plan Part 1

Meaningful Living Plan Part 2

To-Do List

This is Me

Monthly Personal Reflection

Meeting-Agenda

Meeting Minutes

Activity Person of the Month

Feedback Form

Activity Description

Risk Assessment

INTERACTION RECORD SHEET

NAME... ROOM No;............

ACTIVITY UNDERTAKEN/DECLINED 1:1.... GROUP.... DATE....................

OUTCOME

LED BY..

ACTIVITY UNDERTAKEN/DECLINED 1:1.... GROUP.... DATE....................

OUTCOME

LED BY..

CARE PLAN UPDATE

NAME.. ROOM NUMBER..................

DATE	UPDATE	NAME	SIGN

Plans must be updated in line with Company Policy

MEANINGFUL LIVING PLAN PART 1   Date ....

NAME.. ROOM NUMBER.................

Add as much detail as you can from the resident, family and documents.
Address in the first person

FAMILY

HOMELIFE

HOBBIES

CAREER

FOOD

MEANINGFUL LIVING PLAN PART 2
Dimensions of wellness   Date ....

NAME.. ROOM NUMBER..............

PHYSICAL	SPIRITUAL

INTELLECTUAL	EMOTIONAL

OCCUPATIONAL	ENVIRONMENTAL

SENSORY	SOCIAL

TO DO LIST

ADMISSIONS

This is Me

Photos for Care Plans

Family Photos for a memory book and for on walls in rooms

Email address

Introduce yourself to relatives

If you have a social media page, you need permission from the family to allow you to use their photos. Create a signed document for families to sign if your company doesn't have one

WEEKLY

Contact with residents

Contact with Staff

Check Activity Records are kept up to date and dispense new ones

Print photos of activities for the activity board and send them to social media [providing you have the resident or the family approval]

MONTHLY

Collect and assess activity records. Update files

Update plans in more depth when required

Activity Calendar [*over time, try to get 1-2 months ahead*]

Personal Reflections

Budgeting

Activity Ideas

Risk Assessment checks

Choose an Activity Person of the Month & Present Certificate

[great for motivating staff]

6-8 WEEKS [OR AS STIPULATED]

Residents Meeting *[where appropriate]*

Relatives Meeting

Write up minutes & email to relatives/print for residents

QUARTERLY

Assess individual resident's activity plans

ANNUALLY

Assess all paperwork and update

TO DO LIST

A series of weekly/monthly/annual tasks that need to be undertaken. Always state what the task is and when it is to be completed by

Weekly

Monthly

Annual

This is Me

Current photograph of resident

Date ....

NAME..

ROOM NUMBER.................

I PREFER TO BE CALLED..................................

MY IMMEDIATE FAMILY

PEOPLE WHO ARE IMPORTANT TO ME

MY WORKING LIFE

MY FAVOURITE THINGS TO DO

MY FAVOURITE THINGS TO EAT

MY FAVOURITE THINGS TO DRINK

THINGS I DISLIKE

THINGS I AM ALLERGIC TO

MY HABITS

MY FAVOURITE MEMORIES

THINGS THAT MAKE ME ANGRY OR UPSET

APPEARANCE

MY FAVOURITE TV SHOWS, MUSIC, BOOKS

IMPORTANT DETAILS NOT INCLUDED ABOVE

PLEASE ADD PHOTOS BELOW OR GIVE TO US TO SCAN AND RETURN YOUR ORIGINALS

When complete, please return to the Activities Department

PERSONAL REFLECTION   DATE.......................

It is important to self-assess your capabilities and to see where you can make improvements. By spending a few minutes at the end of the month jotting a few things down, you can see where your strengths and weaknesses are. Never be afraid to ask for the necessary training if you feel it will benefit you and the residents. This is purely for your own development not for the files.

Have you managed to have contact with every resident and facilitate their needs?

Have you built on your relationship with staff?

Have you built on your relationship with families?

What do you feel proud of achieving this month?

Where do you think you need to improve your knowledge?

Notes to self

Meeting Agenda for Curlew House
Relatives Meeting
25/8/2020

Present: Self, Mrs AW, Mr PT, Miss AJ, Mr and Mrs TD
Apologies: Mr TT

List numerical points you wish to discuss

1. Ideas for the Christmas Fete

2. Improvements within the home

3. Purchase of Minibus

4. Fundraising

5. Any other business

Allocate someone to take the minutes as it is very difficult to chair a meeting, respond and take notes. Delete the sample elements and use as a template

Minutes of the Meeting on 25/08/2020
for Curlew House
Relatives Meeting

Present: Self, Mrs AW, Mr PT, Miss AJ, Mr and Mrs TD
Apologies: Mr TT

6. Ideas for the Christmas Fete
   Tombola, raffle, lucky dip, weight of the cake
   Action Mr PT

7. Improvements within the home
   New carpets in entrance

8. Purchase of Minibus
   Just Giving Page, fundraising events, sponsorship
   Mrs AW

9. Fundraising

10. To be discussed at next meeting

11. Any other business
    Toiletries Miss AJ

Next Meeting 25/09/2020

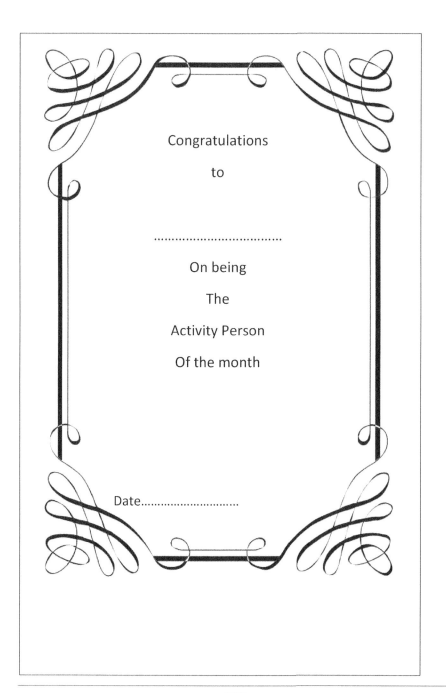

Congratulations

to

....

On being

The

Activity Person

Of the month

Date............................

RESIDENTS AND RELATIVES FEEDBACK

We welcome any feedback from you to help us grow

Are you happy with the meaningful activities we deliver?

Is there anything you would like us to do in particular?

Is there anything you dislike?

Would you be willing to help when we have events and social gatherings like fundraising?

If so, what role would you like to be involved in?

Do you have any ideas for fund raisers that we could develop?

Thank you for your time, please return this to myself or the Administrator.

It would help if you left your details below so we can contact you

Name…………………………………………….. contact No…………………………………………

ACTIVITY DESCRIPTION

NAME OF ACTIVITY ....

DETAILS OF ACTIVITY

EQUIPMENT REQUIRED

GROUP.......... 1:1............. DURATION...

EXPECTED OUTCOME

ACTIVITY RISK ASSESSMENT

ACTIVITY

```
┌─────────────────────────────────────────────────────┐
│                                                       │
│                                                       │
│                                                       │
│                                                       │
└─────────────────────────────────────────────────────┘
```

HAZARD

```
┌─────────────────────────────────────────────────────┐
│                                                       │
│                                                       │
│                                                       │
│                                                       │
└─────────────────────────────────────────────────────┘
```

RISK

```
┌─────────────────────────────────────────────────────┐
│                                                       │
│                                                       │
│                                                       │
│                                                       │
└─────────────────────────────────────────────────────┘
```

HIGH..................... MEDIUM..................... LOW.......................

PRECAUTIONS IN PLACE

```
┌─────────────────────────────────────────────────────┐
│                                                       │
│                                                       │
│                                                       │
│                                                       │
└─────────────────────────────────────────────────────┘
```

REVIEW DATE..

Risk assessment checked by name.. Date...................

Activity	Describe the component parts of your activity
Hazard	List things you anticipate may cause harm or things associated with your activity that have the potential to cause harm
Risk	Assess the risk as either H, M or L when concluding your assessment considering all the circumstances
Precautions	Consider what you might do to minimise/negate the risks
In place	Will the precautionary measures be in place at the time of the activity
Review Date	When would it be reasonable to review your assessment
Reviewer	Name of the person responsible for completing the risk assessment

Chapter 27 **Links**

Dementia UK https://www.dementiauk.org/for-professionals/free-resources/life-story-work/?gclid=Cj0KCQiAmsrxBRDaARIsANyiD1p0yQqkkrzhWXZqTSXG9TqVMX6btWRVwr2XQiPEQzJ9NSNbQ2DAU3AaAmIjEALw_wcB

Thompson R. (2011) Using life story work to enhance care. Nursing Older People 23 (8): 16-21

Alzheimer's UK https://www.alzheimers.org.uk/

Joyce Simard https://www.amazon.co.uk/Namaste-Care-People-Kendall-Nicola/dp/1785928341/ref=pd_sbs_14_img_0/261-6027048-5382038?_encoding=UTF8&pd_rd_i=1785928341&pd_rd_r=a7845c1e-aa3c-4037-974c-cf266dd9940d&pd_rd_w=2eTnb&pd_rd_wg=a1feT&pf_rd_p=e44592b5-e56d-44c2-a4f9-dbdc09b29395&pf_rd_r=11GCRB4EMFDT2T9Q229B&psc=1&refRID=11GCRB4EMFDT2T9Q229B

Worcester University
https://www.worcester.ac.uk/about/academic-schools/school-of-allied-health-and-community/allied-health-research/association-for-dementia-studies/ads-research/current-projects.aspx

Future Learn https://www.futurelearn.com/

Moot https://www.utas.edu.au/wicking/understanding-dementia

PAT Dogs https://petsastherapy.org/

Arts Uplift https://www.artsuplift.co.uk/suitcase-stories-2-can-start/

CQC	https://www.cqc.org.uk/what-we-do/how-we-do-our-job/ratings
NAPA	https://napa-activities.co.uk/services/training

At any time, anything you do must adhere to the law and your company Policies and Procedures

If in doubt, ask!

I hope you have expanded your knowledge by reading this book and have found a few new ways to make your job role easier.

I'm happy to email out A4 templates, drop me a line at

activitieshandbook@outlook.com

Follow us on
https://www.facebook.com/activityhandbook

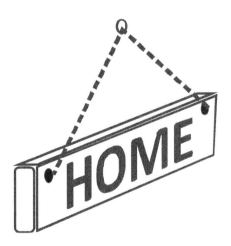

Printed in Great Britain
by Amazon

86353937R00081